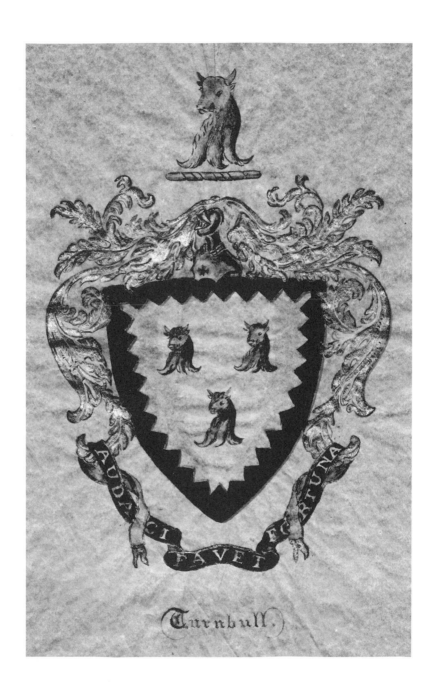

AUDACI FAVET FORTUNA

Turnbull.

THE EXCEPTIONAL LIFE OF JAY TURNBULL

Disability and Dignity in America, 1967–2009

THE EXCEPTIONAL LIFE
OF
JAY TURNBULL

Disability and Dignity in America
1967–2009

RUD TURNBULL

Design by Lynne Adams, Lisa Carta
Offset printed and bound in the United States of America

ISBN 978-0-9662602-9-8
Library of Congress Control Number 2011924983

WHITE POPPY PRESS
34 Main Street
Amherst, Massachusetts 01002
www.whitepoppypress.com
413-253-2353

White Poppy Press is an imprint of Modern Memoirs Publishing

In memory of Jay Turnbull

For Ann, Jay's fiercely devoted mother and visionary, and my beloved wife

*For Amy and Kate, his sisters, who gloried in his life, loved him,
and were loved by him*

With gratitude to all who dignified Jay

With hopes for all who seek rights and dignity in a world of disability

The Jay Turnbull Fellowship

If you benefit from reading this memoir, you may want to consider making a tax-deductible contribution to the **Jay Turnbull Fellowship**, which honors him and supports the education and research of doctoral students at **The Beach Center on Disability**, where Jay worked for 21 years and which Ann and I co-founded and still co-direct.

You may contribute by designating your gift for the Jay Turnbull Fellowship, making it payable to **Kansas University Endowment Association**, and sending it to me at 730 New Hampshire Street, Suite 3K, Lawrence, Kansas, 66044. I will forward it to the Endowment Association.

None of your gift will be used for administrative purposes; all of it will benefit recipients of the Jay Turnbull Fellowship.

If you have questions about the Beach Center, the Jay Turnbull Fellowship, or this memoir, you may email me at Rud@ku.edu. Please enter "Jay Turnbull Exceptional Life" in the title of your email. I will respond as soon as I can.

Thank you.
Rud Turnbull

Archives

The Archives of The University of Kansas contain almost all of the records Ann and I have maintained about Jay. They are histories of my son and our family's "cause" and of the field of intellectual and related developmental disabilities in the years between Jay's birth and death, 1967–2009.

CONTENTS

Introduction

How can it be that a man with multiple disabilities became a man of national significance? A man who had an intellectual disability, autism, rapid-cycling bipolar disorder, and obsessive-compulsive behaviors, and, as an adult, irregular heart rhythms (atrial fibrillation)—such a man was hardly likely to have inspired families and professionals, to have been an impetus in a civil rights movement, to have shaped the lives of parents who had six degrees between them, and to have imbued two sisters with extraordinary compassion.

Yet, when this man, our son, Jay, died on January 7, 2009, at age 41, hundreds of letters from people around the world repeated the same themes: Jay inspired people. Jay gave people hope. Jay showed a new way.

How can that have been? It is because of Jay himself. He insisted on living *his* way and on expecting that by loving others, he would receive their love and support.

There is an imperfect chronology to this memoir. It seemed to me that I could more fully portray Jay and the essence of the meaning of his life if I included information and reflections that do not simply follow a timeline.

Thus, Part I, "Birth and Early Education," is chronological, bringing Jay from his birth to age twenty (1967–1988). Part II, "The Man Himself," tells about Jay himself, ages 21 through 41 (1988–2009). Part III, "Making It in America," turns to themes, describing how he lived a life of dignity, an enviable life, during the last two decades of his life.

Part IV, "Death," begins before Jay died and concludes two years later, to the very day. I leave the narrative style behind and inadvertently plunge into verse, a new form for me. Starting off with my prescience of death and the weekend before Jay died, the first few chapters cover the last days of his life. I try to describe the days immediately thereafter—visitation, funeral, celebration of life, and burial—and then our family's life for the next six months or so.

Part IV cannot, however, begin to tell what Jay's death meant to me and my family. Facts are important but insufficient to describe fully the reality of Jay's cataclysmic death.

So, Parts V and VI expose my bereavement process. The writing is brutally self-reflective. It tells, as honestly as I can write, what happened to me and, to a lesser degree, to Ann, Amy, and Kate, in the two years after Jay died. The verses in these chapters appear in the order in which I wrote them. That fact explains the back-and-forth-ness of the content—the absence of any single narrative, but the presence of many different ones.

Most of the chapters in Part V are laments—my confrontations with grief. Some are verbal wrestling matches with God— arguments that ultimately resolve themselves only through faith. Some affirm the elegant mysteries of life as evidenced by the spontaneous and always timely appearances of symbols. These chapters are about grief, God, and gratitude.

Part VI consists of verses in a different voice. In them, I describe how this person I know so well, this Rud Turnbull, sees himself from afar, bound by grief, struggling with faith, finding reasons for gratitude, and, in the end, comforted by love. Here, he—the author—follows an arc toward peace.

The Postscript briefly describes the public policy contexts in which Jay lived and my role in them, a role that Ann always also carried out as my professional partner and Jay's mother. It makes the point that Jay was our best professor and the catalyst for our professional lives.

There are lessons here for any reader, but this is a memoir, not a textbook, and a reader must derive personal meaning and applicability solo. Of course, this is a book about Jay. But it is equally a book about Ann, Amy, Kate, and me, individually and collectively. Our roles were to bring joy into his life by loving him, all of him, all of the goodness and sweetness and all of the challenges his disabilities created; to support him to become the person he was meant to be and to have the life he wanted to have; and to tell his story.

Here is my memoir of my son. Ann has contributed to it, making my memories more factual and softening my tone and, most importantly, allowing me the solitude to write and being my most comforting companion, my partner, and my beloved not just in the writing about Jay but, foundationally, in being his mother. Without her and without Amy and Kate, the zest-givers in my dark days and my rewards of parenthood, Jay would have never had a life of such dignity, nor I a life so encircled by the dance of love. But the words here are mine, and omissions and errors of fact and judgment are mine and mine alone.

Rud Turnbull
Lawrence, Kansas
December, 2010

ACKNOWLEDGEMENTS

I am grateful for the contributions to this memoir from Lois Weldon, Julie Ann Cisz, Fred and Susan Irons, Peter Luckey, Ruth Luckasson, Holly Riddle, Ann Davis, and Alison de Groot and Lynne Adams of White Poppy Press, publisher.

I am inexpressibly grateful to Ann for her unstinting support of my effort to describe Jay's life and the effects of his death, and for my daughters Amy and Kate, who, typically and jointly, said, "Go for it, Old Bull!"

More than any other person inside or outside our family, Ann envisioned Jay's life of dignity and, in thousands of great and small ways, persuaded others to subscribe to her vision and then to enliven it. Amy, Kate, and I were with her all the way, not always at her side, for she sometimes took larger paces than we could manage—but always in support of her and thus of Jay.

CHRONOLOGY

June 24, 1967   Jay is born at Johns Hopkins Hospital, Baltimore. My ex-wife's parents and large family live in Baltimore. So does my mother, Ruth, and many of my cousins. My father, Henry, lives in New York City. So does my brother John; he marries Silvia Garcia. I am practicing law, first with a big firm and then with a small one.

Summer, 1967–Summer, 1969   I enter Harvard Law School, fall, 1968, earn my masters of law degree, graduate in June 1969, and, with my ex-wife, move to Chapel Hill, North Carolina.

Summer, 1969–Summer, 1972   Jay attends the Sarah Barker Center, Durham, North Carolina, 1969–1970. Evelyn Taylor directs the school; Cordelia Bethea works there. Jay lives with Cordelia, winter, spring and summer, 1974.

Summer/Fall, 1972–August, 1974   I place Jay at Pine Harbor Nursery, Pascoag, Rhode Island. Sister Mary Howard directs the school. Katie McCarthy, age 16 or 17, is a volunteer. She and her family take Jay into their family on weekends and holidays.

Phil Roos, executive director, National Association for Retarded Children, and Paul Marchand, executive director, NARC of Northern Rhode Island, cause the school to be closed. Paul later becomes one of my very best friends and a policy-advocate mentor.

Jay moves from Pine Harbor School to Crystal Springs Nursery, Assonet, Massachusetts. Sue and Dom are the resident staff in Jay's home there. Grandmother Bartlett is Sue's mother.

March, 1974   Ann and I marry. Her father is Hubert Fulton Patterson, known as "A-Dad." Her mother, deceased, is Mary Katherine Boone. Her sister is Virginia (known as "Teo"). She is married to William. They have two sons, Thad and Pate.

August, 1974–August, 1987   Ann and I bring Jay home to Chapel Hill, to be our first child, August, 1974.

May 13, 1975   Amy Patterson Rutherford Turnbull is born.

March 30, 1978   Katherine Cansler Turnbull is born.

August, 1974–August, 1980   Carolyn and Steve Schroeder are Ann's colleagues and become our friends.

Dot and Jim Cansler become Amy's adoptive grandparents and Kate's namesake.

Jay's teachers are Barbara Smith, Roger Moser, Beth McGowan, Frances Hargraves, Randi Silver, and Julie Wong.

Bill Creech is a state senator for whom I drafted the state's special education law.

Al Abeson and Fred Weintraub are colleagues, at the Council for Exceptional Children, with whom I draft the due process regulations implementing the federal special education statute, enacted in 1975.

Summer, 1987   Ann and I admit Jay to the residential services of the local agency for adults. He lives there for a short while and then leaves.

Ann and I create Full Citizenship, Inc.

August, 1987   Ann and I take sabbatical to Washington, D.C. and live in Bethesda, Maryland. Nancy Hickham joins us to assist with our three children.

August, 1987   Jay enrolls in Walt Whitman High School. His teacher is Mary Morningstar.

December, 1987   Jay receives his letter jacket from the tri-captains of the Walt Whitman High School football team.

June, 1988   Jay graduates from Walt Whitman High School, Bethesda.

June, 1988   Jay returns to Lawrence. Chuck Rhodes takes him to the gym and to the SAE fraternity house. Jay meets Pat Hughes and Corey Royer. Pat and Corey create a new university extracurricular entity, "Natural Ties." Jay is the first "tie"—a person with a disability. He is the inspiration for this student organization.

June, 1989   Together with the trustees of a trust created by my ex-wife's parents for Jay's benefit, Ann and I buy a house for Jay, Pat, and Corey, 1120 Hilltop Drive, Lawrence.

Summer, 1989   Jay begins the first in a long succession of housemates:
1989   Pat Hughes and Corey Royer
1989–1991   Jesus and Shala Rosales, joined later by Corey Royer
1993   Tom Allison and Lillie Cusick
1994   Tom Allison, Elizabeth Giffin, and Greg Austin
1995   Tom Allison, Elizabeth Giffin, and Karim Jibril
1996   Karim Jibril, Tim Brown, and Brian Schwegman
1997   Richard Gaeta and Anne Guthrie
2001   Tom and Laura Riffel
2002–2005   Bryan Riffel
2005–2009   Tom and Laura Riffel

August, 1989   Jean Ann Summers, Dick Schiefelbusch, and Ed Zamarripa arrange for Jay to work at KU, assigned to the Beach Center on Disability, which we created in June 1988.
      Within the community, he receives support from staff at Full Citizenship, especially Mary Morningstar, his sisters Amy and Kate, the Natural Ties fraternity-sorority members, and our family's friends.

Mid-summer, early-fall, early winter, 1989-90   Jay, aged 22-23, begins to have a variety of challenging behaviors. Some of these are repeats of behavior he had just after he left New England to be in our family. Some are new. All are more challenging because he is larger and stronger than as a boy and because we do not live with him except on weekends. These behaviors continue throughout his life.

Winter–Spring, 1990   We begin intense and desperate search for help from physicians, especially psychiatrists, psychologists, behavior management specialists, and special educators. We rely on these professionals and Jay's job coaches and co-workers.

Spring–Summer, 1990   Jay begins music therapy. Alice Ann Darrow, a professor at the university, supervises students for nearly 15 years. Other faculty continue her role after she takes a professorship elsewhere.

Jay begins speech-language therapy. Jane Wegner, director of the clinic where graduate students train, supervises students until Jay dies.

Sometime in 1992–1993   Jay begins yoga with Karen Seibel, R.N., and massage with Todd Wyant, C.M.T., and continues these activities until he dies.

1999   The trustees of a trust for Jay's benefit and Ann and I sell the house on Hilltop Drive and buy the house at 1617 Alabama Street, Lawrence. It is Jay's home until he dies.

June 24, 2007   Jay has his 40th birthday party. Nearly 100 guests celebrate it with him.

January 7, 2009, a Wednesday   Jay dies.

January 7 and 8, Thursday and Friday   Amy and Rahul, and Kate and Chip arrive; so do Ann's sister Virginia and her husband, William, our daughters' adoptive grandmother and godmother, Dot Cansler, and our family friends Fred and Susan Irons. The Riffles and Turnbulls select urns and a coffin.

January 8, Friday   Jay's friends visit us and view him at Warren McElwain Funeral Home. There are at least 150 visitors. As befits Jay, we serve food, non-alcoholic drinks, and wine.

January 9, Saturday   Jay's funeral is at Plymouth Church in the morning. The sanctuary is full, some 700 people mourning him and comforting us. That night, nearly 150 family and friends gather for dinner and a celebration of Jay's life.

January 10, Sunday   Jay is buried in Pioneer Hill Cemetery, Lawrence. Amy, Kate, Ann, our Pastor Peter Lucky, Tom and Laura Riffel, and I attend.

April 19, Sunday   Jay's small urn is buried at Prospect Hill Cemetery, Towson, Baltimore County, Maryland. Ann and I attend, together with the gravedigger and cemetery manager.
    Jay's name is inscribed into the Turnbull Family Headstone, winter, 2009.

June 24, 2009   Jay's 42nd birthday, Amy and Kate take us to the planting of a tree to memorialize Jay, and approximately ten friends gather to sing "Happy Birthday, Dear Jay."

September 7, 2009   Nine months after Jay dies, Ann and I witness the installation of the monument at the Jay Tree.

PART I

Birth, Infancy, and Early Education

1
Confronted by Disability: Jay's Infancy

I had not known about disability before Jay was born. I had grown up in a segregated world. In my hometown, Bronxville, New York, restrictive covenants barred sales of homes to African Americans, Asians, and Jews. When I prepared for college at Kent School, a boys' Episcopal school in Connecticut, when I attended Johns Hopkins University, and when I did my graduate work at Maryland and Harvard law schools, academic excellence was the norm and precluded disability. My world had been hugely segregated. Jay's birth banished segregation and immediately required me to confront disability.

Birth and the Days After

It is late on a Saturday afternoon, June 24, 1967. My ex-wife labors at home. She can not wait any longer to go to the hospital; as she enters our car, her water breaks. I drive furiously from our home in north Baltimore, through east Baltimore, flashing the car's lights, honking its horn, weaving in and out of traffic, breaking through stop signs and stop lights, and finally arriving at Johns Hopkins Hospital's emergency room. Nurses take her into the labor room. Her parents arrive, as does her doctor, late to his duties. Jay is born soon thereafter.

Jay lies in a crib in the newborn nursery. There is something especially notable below his blond curls. It is his fontanel. It is convex, not concave, a lump half the size of an egg, protruding. His head, too, is different, significantly out of proportion to his body.

I do not know what to make of these oddities; babies and I are strangers. But I do know there is something different about Jay, something that no one has yet explained.

The Hopkins physicians measure the circumference of his head, not once but often. They proclaim his head size to be "high normal." They deny the possibility of disability. But they do not dispel my doubts and fears.

Weeks go by rapidly. Jay has projectile vomiting; he is floppy in my arms. He and I go to his physician weekly. At every visit, his pediatrician measures Jay's head and tests his strength, looking for signs of normal development. Finally, he admits that Jay has a disability. He does not specify the nature of it, nor its cause. He leaves me puzzled, in a mental and emotional limbo.

I cannot remember whether I asked what I should do for Jay, but I cannot forget the advice I received. It was typical of the advice given in those days to the parents of other children with obvious disabilities, "You should place Jay into an institution."

More than any metric of head size or developmental delay, this advice conclusively warns me that I face a different life than I had ever contemplated.

The pediatricians and neurologists confer and determine that Jay has hydrocephalus, "water on the brain." The water caused him to have convex fontanel and an enlarged head. It also caused him to have the obvious developmental disabilities—floppiness and lack of muscle control and inability timely to achieve developmental milestones. His doctors say Jay needs to have a shunt implanted, and I consent. I am less puzzled about Jay than about his future and mine. I understand about the surgery but I cannot fully take in the concept of disability, much less the advice to institutionalize my son.

On the day of the operation, I await the surgeon; he is hours late. I confront him, asking why the wait. "I've been saving someone's life, Mr. Turnbull, and now I'm about to help your son."

That is a sufficient answer; he has the reputation of having the fastest and best knife at Hopkins.

Jay receives his shunt. It comes too late; Jay's brain is already damaged. My puzzlement grows. Ambiguity about the future becomes constant, but, as questions compound themselves, my commitment to Jay does, too, in inverse relationship.

Early Intervention

Months pass and Jay, now just over a year old, is ready for early intervention. At his physician's suggestion, my ex-wife and I take Jay to the Kennedy Institute, an affiliate of the Hopkins medical institutions. There, Jay and we undergo extensive screenings and evaluations.

A social worker tells us to get a station wagon because Jay will never walk, and we will need a more accessible vehicle than our Chevrolet coupe.

Pediatricians and neurologists recommend intervention designed to elicit responses from Jay. We accede and I weekly take Jay to a psychologist. I observe from the other side of a two-way mirror, watching.

The expert holds Jay on his lap, and offers a banana. Jay reaches for it. The man turns off the room lights and tells Jay, "Say 'ah'." If Jay were to comply, Jay would get another bite of banana. But Jay is silent, or screams.

Time and again, the stimulus-response exercise is repeated. Time and again, I see Jay fail. These days are omens, though I do not know it at the time.

Jay is "non-compliant" at Kennedy, but not with my mother. During his infancy and first three years, he and she sit together, he in her lap, and sing. Mother chooses "Bye Bye Blackbird," and Jay responds, flapping his hands in time with the rhythm and purring the tune. Mother smiles broadly; Jay mimics her. Here, too, is a sign for the future, though, again, I am unaware of it.

2

Jay's Early Childhood

It is now the summer of 1968. Jay is a year old. Having graduated with honors and as editor-in-chief of the law review at the University of Maryland Law School and having clerked for the chief judges of the city and federal courts, I find myself incapable of practicing law. I have no interest in my business or in protecting their clients' already great wealth, nor any taste for the cut-throatedness of my associates and many members of the Baltimore bar.

The Baltimore race riots of 1967, coupled with my failure as a practitioner and my sense that Jay was putting me onto a different path than I had expected, push me out of Baltimore. I matriculate at Harvard Law School in August, 1968, seeking to earn my post-graduate law degree and then find a way to use the law for social good.

My ex-wife refuses to accompany me. She has chronic mental illness and wants the support of her family, and I know she is right to have it. While I am at Harvard, she gives Jay to two of her friends to care for him for a few months while she recovers from her present struggle with her illness. I cannot know it at the time, but the informal foster-care with those friends is the first of several displacements that

Jay will experience.

I commute between Boston and Baltimore for the entire academic year, scheduling classes to start on Mondays and end on Thursdays, reserving Fridays and the weekends to be at home and to see Jay and my ex-wife.

I receive and accept an offer to be assistant professor at the Institute of Government, University of North Carolina, Chapel Hill. My ex-wife and I sell our home, ship our furniture to Chapel Hill, and drive south. I am hopeful for my career and marriage and relieved that I am escaping the disappointed expectations of family in Baltimore and the history of my recent failure as a lawyer.

Driving through Virginia and into North Carolina in June, 1969, seeing the tall loblolly pine trees and creeping kudzu along the sides of Interstate 85, I have a sense that freedom awaits me in this foreign place, this old south, that my family have a chance for a new start in life. Events prove me to be both wrong and right.

Private Charity

There is no school for two-year-old Jay in Chapel Hill, but a day-care nursery in Durham agrees to accept him. I drive him there every morning, and bring him home every night, ten miles one way, ten back. In spring and summer, I take down the top of my convertible automobile, and Jay and I delight in the wind in our hair. I have no idea what the staff should do for Jay, or who the staff are, other than Evelyn Taylor, the director. The professionals are young white women and the aides are older African American women.

Jay is content, still unable to stand, still non-verbal. But the physical world is his to enjoy—wind in his hair, women's arms around him, his father present.

My work requires me to travel throughout the state. Mrs. Taylor knows this; I tell her that I wonder how I can care for Jay when I am traveling, for my ex-wife is hospitalized from time to time. The day after I tell her my predicament, Mrs. Taylor offers an answer. "Cordelia wants Jay. She wants to take him home and care for him, for as long as you need. She loves him. "

I meet Cordelia Bethea formally for the first time. She is married and has children of her own. I look into her eyes and see how she holds Jay, and I say "yes," desperate, having no other choice, and instinctively trusting her. She takes Jay in, this oversized African American woman whose home I never saw.

There are no background checks, no formal assurances and contracts, simply Mrs. Taylor's vouching for her, my desperation to find a home for Jay to substitute for the one I cannot provide, and Jay's sinking comfortably into Cordelia's embrace. Cordelia's race and mine are irrelevant.

Searching

I know I must choose between keeping Jay at home or with Cordelia. If I chose to keep Jay in North Carolina with Cordelia or in my own home with support, I undoubtedly will make it difficult for my ex-wife to leave the hospital. But I believe I must satisfy her needs, so I begin to search for a place for Jay. It is the spring and summer of 1970.

I scour books cataloguing private residential facilities. I visit many public and private institutions, traveling to South Carolina, Pennsylvania, Connecticut, Rhode Island, and Massachusetts, but, on the advice of my ex-wife's father, avoiding public and private institutions in North Carolina and Maryland.

I see children and adults with greatly macrocephalic heads, some with their spinal cords distended, most in cribs covered with mesh that entraps them, others non-ambulatory and in wooden wheel chairs or sitting and rocking on benches.

In their near-nakedness, they seem so unlike Jay, so physically deviant. Some have their limbs restrained by sturdy sail-cloth wraps. When they make noises, they create a cacophony of grunts and wails. Some urinate and defecate where they sit, not on toilets but on metal benches atop floors graded to allow their waste to flow into a hole in the floor; attendants hose them down.

In one private facility, in Belmont, North Carolina, I meet the Roman Catholic Sister in charge; she holds a baby with a hugely distended spinal cord, and speaks softly about God's children and her mission. I make a note: There must be other people like her, somewhere else. I detect the kind of "place" I want for Jay, not that I want any place at all. I want him home. But that is not to be.

I learn about the Pine Harbor Nursery, in Pascoag, Rhode Island, a "home" operated by Roman Catholic nuns. I visit it and meet with Sister Mary Howard, see the children to whom she and other Sisters have committed their lives, meet one or two of the nuns, and ask, "Will you take my son?" She agrees.

Placing

Traveling north with Jay, I stop in Baltimore to let my mother—whom he will later name "Grandmommie Ruthie"—say goodbye to Jay. He is oblivious of the nature of this journey, this diaspora. He sits in her lap, my mother sings, and Jay smiles and giggles. "Bye Bye Blackbird" is her song of choice. It seems both so fitting and so inapposite: "Shut the doors and dim the lights" goes one verse, "I'll be home late tonight." There will be no returning home, none I can foresee. Ahead, there is only an indefinite separation from Jay. Mother and I weep together, sharing a common sorrow.

I arrive at Pine Harbor Nursery and hand Jay to Sister Mary Howard. I kiss him and then, against all my instincts, surrender him to her. He screams, reaches out to me, and torques himself toward

10

me. I flee, refusing, for his sake and mine, to prolong this horrible moment. I am numb; for the first time, I am without Jay. It is late summer, 1970. Jay is just a few months more than three years old. This is the worst day of my life.

Katie McCarthy and Christmas

I am barred from seeing Jay for six months; this is the mandatory "adjustment" time for him. Fall has arrived, Thanksgiving has come and gone, and Christmas approaches.

I receive a telephone call from Sister Mary Howard.

"One of our young volunteers has fallen in love with Jay. She takes him to her home on weekend days, and Jay has captivated her and her family. It's the McCarthy family. Katie wants to know if it is okay to have Jay be Baby Jesus in the community Christmas pageant. He has such lovely blond curls."

I consent, grateful that Jay has a home and is beloved. I am not faithless but cannot divine the future. It is enough to know that some people believe that Jay has a touch of divinity to him.

Nearly two years after Jay dies, Katie learns he is dead and writes. She tells of the day he took his first steps independently: "…he trusted [me and my mother] enough to let go of our hands. He was so proud of himself as he flapped his little hands and crossed his eyes with every step he took after that. Jay brought a lot of joy to our home."

And she tells about his first words:

"One particular Saturday, we were all riding in the car, Jay was sitting on my mom's lap in the front seat, you could do that back then, and we passed a farm. My mother pointed out the cows to Jay and he repeated the word 'cow.' We were all so excited that my dad just kept driving looking for all of the cows in northern Rhode Island. I think that ride lasted at least two hours."

Katie concludes by telling us she is a registered nurse supporting adults with developmental disabilities, in Massachusetts:

"So you see, Jay had a life long effect on me and I believe I am a better person for having known and loved Jay Turnbull if only for a short time. There will always be a very special place in my heart for Jay where he continues to giggle and cross his eyes."

Summer comes and I visit Jay for the first time in six months. His crib is in a room with other children's beds and cribs. Upon seeing me, Jay tries to climb out of his crib. One of the Sisters restrains him until I lift him out and hold him tightly.

We stay that way for hours, locked into our desperate embrace. The visit ends just before dinner is served, and I offer Jay, once again, to Sister Mary Howard.

Jay grabs my hair and will not let go; he has found a purchase, not my clothes but my body itself, and he will not release me. He yells as I disentangle his hands from my hair. I rapidly leave the room, and his screams follow me. They mimic his screams of six months ago; nothing has changed—Jay and I are still separated and he painfully knows it.

The summer of 1971 comes and I return to Pine Harbor. Jay, four years old, still cannot walk far without support. And he cannot speak an intelligible sentence.

But he surprises me as I push him in a stroller around the school grounds: He begins to sing, a small, tiny sound, tinny and reedy, the words barely detectable. I stop pushing him, kneel to face him, and listen carefully. "Michael, row your boat ashore," he sings.

His pitch is solid; he is speaking, making words for the first time in his life.

These first words, put to music, clue me about him, though I do not yet know the meaning of the clue, only that he can communicate. I join him in song, crying joyfully.

Only later do I discern the meaning of the clue and significance of "Michael." It is simply this: Jay, joy, music, and communication are inseparable.

Phil Roos and Paul Marchand, who would become my colleagues and, in Paul's case, one of my closest friends, visit Pine Harbor, acting on behalf of the Rhode Island Association for Retarded Children. They notify state and local authorities that the school violates fire and other safety codes. The state orders the school to close. It is late summer, 1971.

Sister Mary Howard calls me after finding another school for Jay, this one nearby, in Assonet, Massachusetts. "I have arranged for Jay to be admitted and will take him there myself. Trust me, Jay will be fine." She has cared for Jay as much as for me; she overwhelms me with her grace.

In the early fall, I visit Jay at the Crystal Springs Nursery in Assonet, meet the director, and confer with the medical director. I later become his colleague in a professional association. He is Allen Crocker, professor of pediatrics at Harvard Medical School.

I also meet Jay's new "parents," for Jay has been moved from the main dormitory to a group home operated by the school. They are Sue and Dom, and they live in the community, where Sue's mother, "Grandmother Bartlett" also lives. They bring Jay into their home. My mother and I visit them, grateful for their giving such compassionate care to Jay, and happily receiving their assurances of his well-being.

I am learning lessons—first taught by Sister Mary and Katie McCarthy and now by Sue, Dom, and Grandmother Bartlett—about shaping Jay's life around the stability that only a family can give. Not my family, for my wife and I are headed toward a divorce, but a family, any family.

13

3
"First, We'll Bring Jay Home"

It is late summer, 1972. I have mononucleosis and hepatitis and am on extended sick leave from work. A colleague's wife brings me a book to read—John Fowles' *Magus*. I devour it and, as I close it, I realize I must end the life I am living. There is another reality for me; I must find it. I ask my ex-wife for a divorce; she consents and we part amicably.

I rent an apartment in Durham, bringing with me the hunting-bird prints, desk, and two rugs I had bought. These are the flotsam and jetsam of a failed marriage—these and Jay's uncertain future in New England. The summer of 1972 is both an end and a beginning. I know what I am leaving. I have no plan for the future and no imagination of it, either.

Separation and divorce suit me. I enjoy myself widely, but briefly and ultimately un-satisfyingly.

In the fall of 1973, Carolyn Schroeder, who had been Jay's psychologist before he left Chapel Hill, acquires a new colleague. She is Ann Patterson.

Ann has moved to Chapel Hill to take up her role as special education director of the Division on Developmental Disabilities at the University of North Carolina. She is recently divorced and asks her colleague Carolyn for suggestions about men to date. Carolyn knows me and suggests that Ann may want to meet me.

Ann acts on Carolyn's suggestion and attends the fall semester organizational meeting of the Orange County (North Carolina) chapter of the Association for Retarded Children (now called The Arc). She enters strategically late—some five to ten minutes after I, as president, have convened the meeting. She sits in the front row, certain to be noticed, and volunteers for every committee for which I seek members. I record her name and number and, with a week, take her for our first date, to the least impressive of all luncheonettes, the Dairy Queen. We drive there in my convertible, its top down, the air messing her carefully arranged hair.

A week or so later, on a proper evening date, we open up to each other, she speaking of her recently deceased mother, I of Jay. We share our sorrows, looking to our pasts but not our futures.

Months later, Ann and I are in her apartment, Jay is "on leave" from Crystal Springs Nursery, and we are considering whether to marry. Ann and I are in the living room. Jay is sitting on the floor of the hallway leading to the back of Ann's apartment.

He begins to sing "Kumbaya," and now for the first time he becomes a medium, for that is the song Ann, her sister, and her father sang at her mother's deathbed, for hours on end, before she died.

Jay, music, and an anthem: I do not pretend to understand what is happening.

On New Year's Eve, 1973, Ann and I return to my apartment from a party at Steve and Carolyn's home. We hold each other, speak of our love and future, and agree to marry.

We marry three months later, but not before Ann tells me,

"First, we'll bring Jay home."

"We'll bring Jay home" is not a matter for discussion; it is a foregone conclusion. We marry, honeymoon at the Schroeders' beach house at Emerald Isle, North Carolina, and, on our return to Chapel Hill, speak about bringing Jay home. We agree to write about bringing people home, and outline our first jointly written article. We conclude the article by arguing it is proper policy to bring all the "Jays" home from institutions.

Ann had worked in one, the Partlow State School and Hospital, in Tuscaloosa, Alabama; I had seen far too many of them during the year I searched for a "placement" for Jay. Our knowledge and our instincts—to have our own family, one that includes Jay—prompts our first co-authored article.

In August, we drive to New England, to bring Jay home. We stop in Baltimore, where I had attended college and law school and practiced law, to meet my mother; in Bronxville, where I had grown up; in Kent, Connecticut, where I boarded in high school; and in Nantucket, Massachusetts, where, in 1944, after my father and mother divorced, mother had taken me and my brother to escape the messiness of the divorce.

I think of Thomas Wolfe's observation, "You can't go home again." But Ann and I are doing just that, retracing my paths into adulthood. Ann becomes pregnant with Amy. Both psychologically and biologically, we are forming our own family.

From Nantucket, we go to Assonet, Massachusetts, the end-stop on our northern journey. There, we bring Jay into our family, physically adding him to the two of us and, unknown to us at that time, to the third of us, Amy, whom Ann carries in her womb.

We had prepared Jay for his homecoming, calling him on the telephone weekly. In each conversation, we would tell him, "We love you, Jay T." And he would respond, his language limited, his words garbled. We hear him speak a word that we understand to be "Portello," and I guess he is referring to an Italian or Portuguese friend. I remind Ann how heavily populated Massachusetts is with Americans whose families came from those countries.

Upon arriving at Sue and Dom's, we meet "Portello." He is Paul Taylor, and he is Jay's age, an African American boy with an Afro. We greet and then take our leave of him and other children: Annie Raffle, Johnny Corkle, Elaine Loomis, and others. (Until the day he died, Jay remembered and prayed for them and for Sue and Dom and Grandmother Bartlett, reminding us nightly that he constituted his family according to the degrees of love, not degrees of kinship.)

Sue and Dom and Grandmother Bartlett bid us farewell, tears in their eyes, for they love Jay. Standing behind them is Paul Taylor, whose farewell to us is the classic "High Five." Jay, a brother to these young people, Jay is going home again.

But to a much different home and to a new mother, for Ann confirms that she will be his mother, as she constantly was each day thereafter. He is seven years old.

Jay is in the backseat of our car, and we are driving southward. He sings, "He's Got the Whole World in His Hands," prophetically musicalizing his reaching out to bring people into his life. He plays with his tinker toys and keeps talking about Portello, over and over again.

Ann tells me, "Turn around, we have to bring Paul Taylor home with Jay." I remind her, we have no authority to do so; bringing him with us is a type of kidnapping, and we have no idea what our future will be.

Law aside, there is another consideration. We are committed to Jay. If we bring Paul Taylor into our family, will we want to have other children, our own biological heirs? We know we want them, so we must leave Paul Taylor behind.

But Jay does not. He continues to talk about Portello, teaching us that race and kinship are insufficient criteria for defining a family.

And when he does not talk about Paul Taylor, he sings, "He's Got the Whole World in His Hands," driving home a lesson about inclusion and blessings.

Throughout his life, he prefers that song to many others, adding other people to a list of remembered people that includes Paul Taylor, Sue, Dom, and Grandmother Bartlett, his former family.

4
Life in the
"Southern Part of Heaven"

Life changes radically after Ann and I bring Jay to live with us in Chapel Hill. Each of us has been single; she had no children from her first marriage; Jay has been in New England for three years and now is in our family. We are naively confident in the future.

Jay's First Lessons as Our Teacher

Jay has been home for about a month, and Ann takes him shopping with her at Sears Roebuck in Durham. He begins to rage, falling to ground, thrashing, yelling, and hitting his head on the floor. Ann does not know how to stop him. She realizes, for the first time, that her training is inadequate.

She earned her doctorate at age twenty-four, specializing in mental retardation, and had taught special education and been a regional consulting specialist in public schools in Georgia. Yet she does not know precisely what to do for and with Jay.

Not for the first time, Jay becomes our teacher: "You have much to learn about why I act this way." Little do we know that these rages will be part of his life until the day he dies.

We cannot understand why he rages, but we hypothesize that he fears abandonment. I recall how he held on to me by grasping my hair when I left him at Pine Harbor Nursery. We do not yet understand that he needs predictability in his daily routine. We do understand, however, that he needs stability in his relationships.

Jay and His Right to an Education

It is now late summer, 1975, and Jay is eight years old, old enough to attend public schools. Ann and I visit with the local school superintendent, and ask for Jay to be admitted to school. He replies, "You first must get a grant from the state department of education and find some teachers. Then, come back and we'll find a classroom for those kids."

We comply, and Jay begins his education, placed into a "classroom" that is in the school district's administrative building. It has been a large storage room and now is the only classroom in the building. His teachers are the well-experienced Frances Hargraves, an African American, and Ann's doctoral and masters' students at the university. Their supervisor is Ann Sanford, one of Ann's professional friends. Like us, they all accept Jay's and their own second-class status and segregation.

I have been working with state senator Bill Creech to draft and secure the enactment by the North Carolina General Assembly of the "Creech Bill," the state's first special education entitlement law. The state law mirrors a model special education law I have researched and written with Fred Weintraub and Al Abeson, the governmental affairs staff at the Council for Exceptional Children.

Further, Congress has enacted P.L. 94-142, the Education for All Handicapped Children Act, providing federal funds to state and local education agencies so they can educate all students with disabilities. Federal courts in Pennsylvania and the District of Columbia, and a state court in Maryland, have held that these children have a constitutional right to a free appropriate public education with children who do not have disabilities. The federal law codifies these decisions.

On the first day of the school year, fall, 1976, Ann and I dress Jay for school and take him to the curb to be picked up by the school bus. The bus, however, does not stop for him. We are in the right place, but we are overlooked and Jay is by-passed.

I go to the local superintendent, pull a copy of the state and federal laws out of my briefcase, and tell him, "The bus had better stop the next morning or I'll sue you and I am the most qualified person in North Carolina to do so."

The next morning, we wait at the curb. The bus stops, and thus begins Jay's right-based education.

Some of Jay's classmates are white, others African American. Most have intellectual disabilities, others have other disabilities, too.

Jay and they have a class in different wing of the elementary school building. At least, we say to ourselves, he has a right to an education, and at least he is not in the administrative building but a real school. We continue to accept the segregation from students who do not have disabilities; we prefer a lesser degree of segregation to a greater one. And we understand how race-based the classification is, not doubting that Jay has a disability but questioning whether some of his classmates—some of the African American students— truly need to be in special education.

Ann reminds me: this is how life is in special education. She has more certainty than I, and more experience with special education segregation, having taught and been a consultant in special education in Georgia and Alabama. Disability congeals people who, in that time and place, rarely would have been together but for that condition.

21

Ann and I cannot accept that discrimination for Jay or others, and we vow to disprove the segregationists. Sadly, we must confront segregation all too often, for Jay is not included—really included in a school—until he is twenty years old. It takes us thirteen years fully to keep our vow. Such is the pace of change; we learn never to overestimate the power of inertia.

Jay and the First Aggression

In summer, 1977, Jay enrolls at a summer camp at a nearby school. It is for students with disabilities. There, he pulls pig-tails of young girl. He has pulled my hair at Pine Harbor. He has pulled Ann's hair. Why?

Throughout most of his life, he seemingly inexplicably pulls people's hair, sometimes grabbing strangers' hair, more often pulling mine, Ann's, and that of the young women we hire to be with him after school adjourns and before we return from work. Years later, as an adolescent and then adult, he pulls the pony-tails of guests at a local restaurant, a cleaning woman at a nursing home, and a young girl who lived down the street from him in Lawrence.

When brought to a summer program in Champaign-Urbana, Illinois, in 1976, he fell to the ground, refusing to move—the classic beached whale—and pulled Ann's hair as she tried to lift him up.

Each time he attacks a stranger, we explain and beg forgiveness; each time, forgiveness is forthcoming. Our greatest fear—Jay trapped in the criminal justice system—never materializes.

We speculate why he aggresses. Is it anger? Fear of loss? Of what? Of the security of family?

Ancient experiences seem to explain present behavior: Jay has lost too many people. The coda to his first family (my first wife and I) was my decision to place him in school in Rhode Island. He has been to and taken away from Sister Mary Howard and Katie

McCarthy at Pine Harbor; and from Sue, Dom, Grandmother Bartlett, and Paul Taylor in Massachusetts.

True, he has a new family: Ann; Amy, born within a year after Ann and I brought Jay home; and Kate, born three years after Amy; and I. But Jay has a remarkable long-term memory; he still prays for these people from New England.

He teaches us a lesson we do not readily learn: Do not leave me. Or, if you do, be sure you leave me with a real family. Years later, we relearn the lesson. Until then, we are Jay's family.

Also, years later, in Lawrence, we add Suzanne Kiper, Natalie Turner, Christie Baugh, Christie Woods, Katie Schwartzburg, and other young women to our family. We begin to build an intentional community, an extended family. Jay has taught us to do so, and his and our daughters' needs and our careers require us to do so.

Jay and the First Community Exclusion

Ann and I work as assistant professors, putting in the long hours necessary to climb the professorial ladders to tenure. Sometimes, we hire child-care workers to come to our home; sometimes, we try to enroll Jay in a child-care program in another family's home.

A colleague tells me that his wife operates a program in their home and asks if we are interested. We speak with the wife and enroll Jay.

Two weeks later, she tells us she cannot accommodate him. He wets his pants six or seven times each day; try as she may, she cannot look after him and other children, who have been toilet trained.

The ability to control the sphincter is the golden-key for admission and retention in programs for children with and without disabilities.

23

Turnbull and Patterson Families

Jay's immediate family are Ann, Amy, and Kate. Jay never knew Ann's mother, Mary Katherine Boone Patterson. She died in 1971, when Jay was in New England and before Ann and I met each other.

He did, however, know my father, but only as a baby and then as a youngster. Dad had visited me in Baltimore in fall of 1967, when Jay was a baby. He was present when Ann and I married, and, after we brought Jay home from Massachusetts, he came to our first home in Chapel Hill in 1975, before leaving the country to work as an advertising consultant in Taiwan. He died in January, 1976, never having seen Jay again.

My mother knew Jay well, both in Baltimore before I moved to Chapel Hill and then when she moved to Lawrence at Thanksgiving, 1988, a few months before she died in February, 1989. They formed a duet whenever they meet, whether in Baltimore or Lawrence. Between them, joy was shared, delight amplified. She grieved when I placed Jay at Pine Harbor Nursery, approved when Ann and I brought Jay home, and accepted Jay as he is but worries about Ann and me and our capacities to raise a family of three children.

My brother John barely knows Jay but regularly expresses his interest in and concern about him. There is no doubt, John would be in Jay's and our corner if there ever were a need for him. So, too, would his son Kenny, a man of great intelligence and kindness.

Ann's father—Hubert Fulton Patterson, known as "A-Dad"—moves to Lawrence in 2000. He has known Jay ever since Ann and I married and he finds his way into Jay's heart, singing "You get a line, I get a pole, we'll go down to the craw-dad hole." Jay mimics A-Dad, striking a wooden match, lighting a pipe, shaking out the match's flame, and tossing it into a metal wastepaper basket. They nap simultaneously and are comfortable with each other.

But A-Dad is not comfortable with Jay's disability. As much as he loves Jay as he is, he thinks there must be a cure. In desperation one day, he looks closely at Jay and turns to us. "You've tried everything, haven't you?"

We are puzzled; his question is out of context. "What do you mean, A-Dad?"

He tells us, "I'm talking about Jay. About the key. There must be a key that unlocks his mind." He does not pause. "Have you considered taking Jay to a faith healer?"

No, we tell him, but we have tried everything else to obliterate Jay's challenging behaviors, and now we take Jay as he is. A-Dad tries, but he is an engineer, a problem-solver, a constructor of new buildings; he fashions structures. That which has been built erroneously can be torn down and rebuilt. He wonders, why can't we repair the faulty part of him?

Just as A-Dad comes into Jay's life, so, too, do Ann's sister, Virginia (nick-named "Teo") and brother-in-law William and their two sons, Thad and Pate. They live in West Point, Georgia, on the Chattahoochee River, and their acceptance of Jay is as natural as the heat of south Georgia and the gentle flow of the river that runs through it. They never refer to Jay's limitations, only to his attractive features and gregarious nature. Teo opens her heart to him; he enters it easily, knowing the authenticity of her love. Thad and Pate delight in his idiosyncracies, Thad's warm heart and Pate's curiosity apparent and welcoming. William is kind and includes Jay in the family's errands and in playing ball with the family's many dogs.

The Cansler and Irons Families: Adoptive Grandparents

We acquire adoptive grandparents in Chapel Hill, but not at our own initiative. Dot Cansler is a social worker in the field of developmental disabilities. She and Ann become friends, sharing a common interest in families, especially those who have children with disabilities. By now, Amy is just over three years old and Kate is not yet born. Dot asks Ann, "I want grandchildren. Is it alright if I become grandmother to Amy?"

Dot bears a remarkable resemblance to Ann's mother, who died two years before Ann and I married. Ann instinctively and immediately says, "Yes."

I am unsure about extended family; I value privacy more than Ann. Dot's husband, Jim, the vice chancellor for student affairs at the university, is also unsure. Our brides prevail.

We formalize this extended family by inviting Dot and Jim to be Kate's godparents, and we name Kate for them: Katherine Cansler Turnbull. Ann's mother is part of Kate, too. Mary Katherine Patterson was her name.

Naming is symbolic. Jay carries a formal name: Jesse Lawrence Turnbull—Jesse is a name within my ex-wife's family, and Lawrence is a Turnbull ancestor. Naming honors lineage; it acknowledges that family is central. In naming Kate for Dot and Jim and for Ann's mother, we begin to realize: We must create family beyond our own family.

Another family becomes part of our own, also accidentally. Ann prepares for Amy's birth by attending Lamaze classes. She meets Susan Irons; they become fast friends. Susan and Fred, her husband, meet Jay and instantly accept and love him. It is the fall of 1974.

Unspoken among us is a fear that Jay instills: What if our child has a disability? I do not speak of that prospect; the others are silent, too. I cannot read their minds, but I know mine: Is disability a curse, a punishment for all that I should not have done or have left undone?

In time, of course, Jay's disability—which is to say, Jay himself— was the exact opposite of a punishment: he was a gift.

Jim dies in 1999, widowing Dot. She remains a steadfast friend; likewise, Fred and Susan.

Jay's life and Amy's birth brought Dot, Jim, Susan, and Fred to us; Jay's death brings them back to us. Together with Ann's sister Teo and her husband, William, they come to Jay's funeral services. Thad and Pate, Teo and William's children, are unable to attend. Family is forever, and neither blood nor marriage limits its boundaries.

Happy Times, Sad Times

Jay, Ann, Amy, Kate and I have many happy times in Chapel Hill. Our professional friends welcome Jay into their social lives. Strangers smile at him as we walk the downtown streets. He learns the fight song of the university athletic teams, "I'm a Tar Heel Born," and sings it to the delight of those in his company, bringing them together, showing them a common way. He gives a "high five" to everyone he meets, insisting that this handshake, his way, is the only way to encounter him. And he sings for us and our friends, so happily that we usually join him—a chorus of the competent led by a person otherwise not so competent.

There also were sad times—learning his IQ score is in the low- to mid-40s, and being unable to prevent his nascent emotional-behavioral cycle of mania and depression. He breaks the frames of his eyeglasses so often that our optician deeply discounts each new purchase, realizing the drain on our family's finances. He perseverates, repeating the same phrase or request until we respond to him. He has no friends other than his schoolmates and their parents, or the parents of our daughters' friends. He engages in obsessive-compulsive behaviors, insisting that the physical world he occupies be designed to fit his sense of everything in its place. When extremely frustrated, he acts out, injuring himself and striking at us when we try to prevent him from hurting himself. We realize that Jay has two selves—the one so engaging, the other so challenging.

Symbols

Beyond the music in our lives, there are symbols, inexplicable when first encountered but, in time, comprehensible. Two manifest themselves early in our lives with Jay—pipes and tinker toys.

My father dies in January, 1976, succumbing to sclerosis of the liver that manifest his many years as an alcoholic. Ann, Amy, Jay, and I go to Baltimore County, Maryland to bury my father's cremains. We gather with the large Turnbull family and its many friends at my uncle's homestead, "Blackacre," in Sparks, north of Towson.

Ann, Amy, Jay, and I drive to Prospect Hill cemetery, where three generations of my family are buried. We are all silent, alone in our memories of my father, all silent, except Jay.

Dad had been in Taiwan almost a year before he died, and had called me at Christmas season to read me a parody of the song, "On the First Day of Christmas." It is ribald, and Dad delighted in it.

On the way from Uncle John's to the cemetery, Jay begins to sing, "On the First Day of Christmas." Then, "My eyes have seen the glory of the coming of the Lord," from "The Battle Hymn of The Republic." Then, "Kumbaya."

Jay channels our ancestors.

We stand at the family plot. A soft snow falls. Someone places the urn containing my father's ashes into the ground and covers it with the removed sod. A priest prays from the Episcopal Church's Book of Common Prayer. Ann holds Amy; Jay stands beside me, one hand in mine, the other grasping his tinker toys.

He releases my hand, walks to my father's grave, and places his tinker toys on the grave. He says, "Granddaddy Turnbull is in Heaven with Baby Jesus, smoking a pipe."

When Jay dies thirty-three years later, we place tinker toys in his casket; he takes them to Granddaddy Turnbull.

It is nearly six months later, Sunday, July 4, 1976. We learn that tinker toys are more than symbols.

Ann, Amy, and I are traveling from Chapel Hill to Champaign-Urbana to teach at the University of Illinois. Jay, in the back seat of our car with Amy, has been patient during the two days' journey, but his patience runs out as we enter Champaign-Urbana. "Tinker toys," he repeats time and again; he becomes agitated, and we fear he will have another rage, another episode of aggression or self-injury. We drive around the town, searching for a toy store, desperate to satisfy his need. It seems it takes us forever to find any open store; it is a weekend and national holiday.

We finally succeed and, with relief, buy tinker toys. Jay shapes them into a pipe and "smokes" it. He is at peace. His agitation abates. He has needed reassurances, the familiarity of objects, the solid wood that comforts him and declares that the world is predictable.

Pipes persist in our lives. It is now the first day of August, 1980. We are leaving Chapel Hill for Lawrence and our new professorships at the University of Kansas (KU). Jay, Ann, and I are in our car; Amy and Kate will follow a few days later with Grandmother Dot.

Standing at the front door of our home on North Lake Shore Drive is Steve Schroeder. Carolyn is unable to be there, obliged by duties at work. Jay holds tightly to the corn cob pipe Steve has given him. It is a security object, a reassurance that Steve loves him.

Jay puts the pipe to his mouth and mimics Steve lighting it with the old wooden matches and then shaking out the match. He has perfected these gestures by copying A-Dad. They honor those whom he loves.

Steve weeps; we all do, all except Jay. Does he somehow know that, some fifteen years later, Steve will come to KU, recruited heavily by us and others? Is the pipe a worldly symbol of past and future?

As I clean out his room and closets after he dies, I find a corn-cob pipe. It is too late to put it into his casket. I take it home for keepsake.

I entertain a speculation: Are tinker toys more than reassurances of predictability, and is the pipe more than an artifact of friendship? Are these symbols of Jay's para-normalcy? In time and against all of my training and professional work, I conclude they are. The conclusion seems defensible in light of yet more symbols— butterflies and blackbirds.

Butterflies

On the day Ann buried her mother, May 1, 1972, in West Point, Georgia, butterflies surrounded her mother's casket and the funeral party. Years later, in 1978, Kate is born.

We bring Kate home, lay her on a blanket that Ann's grandmother Boone had made, and take her photograph. Two butterflies alight on her. Each is colored black and blue, the colors of the Johns Hopkins athletic teams. Hopkins is a family alma mater; most of my male ancestors attended and graduated from it, as I did.

Years pass, I return to Kent School for my 40th reunion, in 1999, and, as we leave the school chapel on Sunday morning to return Kate to New York, butterflies alight in the gardens outside the chapel.

More years pass and it is some weeks after we bury Jay. Ann, Amy, Kate, and I are shopping for coffee in Lawrence. It is still winter, mid-February, 2009. We go to a coffee/kitchen-ware shop. In the window, Ann sees a stained-glass plate, some 5 x 7 inches. In it, there are butterflies, colored blue and black, and, surrounding the butterfly, the letters "JT." We turn the ornament over, and the "JT" becomes "TJ," the name of the dog who lived with him at his home in Lawrence.

The animate butterflies, and the inanimate tinker toys, music, and stained glass link Jay to us and to other family members. What is the true nature of his giftedness, and of his being a gift to us?

5

Community, Failure, and Aspiration

Ann and I have no idea what lies ahead as we leave Chapel Hill for Lawrence, Kansas. I depart from an excellent faculty and many good friends, Ann from a good faculty and fewer good friends. Both of us say goodbye to our dearest friends, Steve and Carolyn Schroeder, Dot and Jim Cansler, and Susan and Fred Irons. We do not know that another friendship awaits us, one as deep and lasting as those we have formed in Chapel Hill.

The Welcome and a Safe Harbor

It is August 3, 1980, a hotter day than I've ever known before. We are moving into our new home. I put our name, Turnbull, on our mailbox.

Less than an hour later, Margaret Ann Schwartzburg walks over from the house next door. She carries a large silver tray, bearing lemonade in a silver pitcher, with silver goblets to serve it from, and cookies. She introduces herself, "My maternal grandmother was Margaret Turnbull Pentland. We are related."

Thus begins a friendship of joy, for Jay always delighted in her embrace, laughter, and graciousness, in her obvious love of him, and her husband David, in his playing "La Bamba" on a tennis racket, dancing with a mop, clowning around all the time. Their daughter Katie becomes the best friend of our daughter Kate. They are so close to each other that we call them "hamburger" and "cheeseburger"— two of the same kind, barely indistinguishable from each other. Jay finds pure acceptance with Margaret Ann and David.

Their daughter Lauri becomes Jay's and our daughters' sitter while we work. Katie takes Jay to lunch every Tuesday during her four years as an undergraduate at KU. For several years after she graduates, her sorority sisters carry on as she did.

Explaining Jay to Other Children

It is 1980 and Amy is five years old, thirteen years younger than Jay. She understands Jay has an intellectual disability and she has already been shaped by him. Her friends, however, do not understand his disability. They do not understand why his head is larger than normal, or why he walks in a funny way. One of her friends asks her, "What's wrong with your brother?" She explains, "Jay's brain is like a record player. It plays music at a slow speed. Our minds play music at fast speeds. But he and we are like each other: we all make music."

A year later, Amy must again answer her friends' inquiries about Jay. Amy explains, "When Jay's mom was pregnant, she fell down the stairs, and it hurt Jay's brain."

We tell her, "That's not true." She answers, "I know, but, you don't understand, little kids can't handle it when you say you don't know why something happened. If you can't give them a reason, they worry 'bout it. It's better to give a reason so they won't have to worry. Can't we just make it easy for them?"

In her elementary school, Amy is required to participate in a science fair. She administers a pre-test to her classmates about mental retardation; she then teaches about it and uses Jay as an example; she then administers a post-test. The results are remarkable: the students' attitudes and knowledge have increased significantly. Amy enters her project into the competition and receives third place. She is disappointed and justifies the result, "The judges must have been Republicans!"

Still in elementary school, she presents a poster-board session at the American Association on Mental Deficiency, of which I am an officer. There, she receives much praise from many people. She hypothesizes that they must be Democrats or, if not, at least more enlightened than some Republicans.

Kate, too, reveals Jay's early influence. She also does research on attitudes, using the pre-test, teach, post-test approach. Her results mimic Amy's. With the assistance of one of our doctoral students, she crafts an article and publishes it. She is only ten years old. Some years later, she is the editor in chief of the Barstow School newspaper and editorializes against the students' use of the word "retard." In the research, she displays her mind; in the editorial, her heart.

Jay's spirit—his seeming ability to transcend the immediate conditions of his life—and his unintentional but consequential contributions to our daughters' hearts are not his only gifts. There is yet another. Not surprisingly, it is spiritual, in the theological sense.

We attend Plymouth Congregational Church, and Amy and Kate enroll in confirmation classes. Each is selected to speak on behalf of their class when confirmed before the congregation. Ann and I do not coach them on what to say, nor do their Sunday school teachers. Each speaks about faith, and each attributes their faith to Jay.

School Days

Jay's first teacher in Lawrence refuses to read Jay's Individualized Education Program (IEP) from Chapel Hill, saying, "I want to know him before I teach him." We accede, but we wonder: Will Jay really benefit from a person who wants to learn it all for herself? How do we create partnerships among independent professionals?

This teacher is kind to Jay and teaches him some skills. Jay fares much worse with his next teacher. She is hostile to us, unwilling to meet to discuss Jay. Jay and we endure her for a year; we fail to change her.

In Jay's second year with that teacher, we resort to a different strategy. One of our colleagues assigns one of our doctoral students to do a practicum in the classroom Jay attends. He asks her to record what she learns, but she takes his request to a different level and keeps a secret notebook, recording what she observes.

At the end of the year, we read the notebook. It is damning. Among other things, it records how the teacher prompted a student with significant intellectual disability to ask for a job from an exhibitor at the school job-fair. The exhibitor turned the student away angrily, with obvious prejudice. Our student has recorded the episode, including the teacher's remark, made as she sent the student to the exhibitor, "Watch that little frog [referring to her student] get thrown back into our pond."

Ann, our student, and I take the book to the school district's special education director. He listens to our student, reads her notebook, and soon thereafter refuses to renew the teacher's contract.

Years later, the state director of special education tells us he has long been puzzled about our response to Jay's obviously inappropriate education. It was not just one teacher who, he knows, has disappointed us and short-changed Jay. Because Jay has been out of school for several years, the man is safe in asking, "Rud, why didn't you simply sue us about that teacher and Jay's poor education?"

I respond, "Because I needed your help, not your animosity. Jay would be in school for many more years. I didn't want to spend them in an adversary relationship with you and I didn't want to risk retaliation against Jay or his sisters or other students with disabilities."

The man nods, silently acknowledging that my reasons were sound.

Jay's education in elementary school is satisfactory, nothing more. His education in high school is deplorable. Day after day, he and his classmates watch TV's *Bill Cosby Show*. Why the show, we ask? "I am teaching them leisure skills," his teacher responds. That, and how to wash the athletic gear of the high school teams, for, of course, the classroom is next to the laundry, separated from the other students, convenient for the menial and low-expectation work that serves others but does not advance Jay's or his peers' abilities.

We learn about low expectations and how hard it will be to instill great expectations in professionals.

Far too often, Jay's teacher telephones me or Ann to ask us to come to school, calm Jay down, or take him home. Clearly, he and she are not suited for each other. She cannot change; neither can he. They are at loggerheads except when she is "teaching" him to watch television or he is washing the athletes' towels. She sees nothing wrong with this "curriculum."

On the Wrong Path

In the 1980s there is but one destination in our community after high school, and it is the group home and sheltered workshop operated by a local agency. The agency has state and local governmental funding; it is well regarded in town. Many of the most powerful people in town serve on its board of directors. It also is the only service agency in town; it has a monopoly.

Jay is now eighteen, and the year is 1985. He has three years of school eligibility left, but he is at the top of the long list of people waiting for admission to the agency's programs. We accept admission, for, we think, there is no other way for Jay and us, and we do not want him to be relegated to the bottom of the waiting list. The waiting list and the monopoly drive our decision. We make the choice: take what we can when we can, however inadequate it is and however much it runs against our ideology of inclusion. But we do more than accede to the ordinary. Ann serves on the agency's board of directors, seeking to reform the agency from within but meeting obstacles and objections to every one of her suggestions for state-of-the-art practice.

Nearly involuntarily—for our choice was services now or none for a long time—we have gone from segregation in Jay's school years to segregation in his adulthood. We find too soon that we have erred gravely.

Yet, from our family's perspective, it is time for Jay to transition from home to congregate care. We are exhausted from advocating for him and caring for him. Our daughters need more of our attention; they have endured his outbursts; they have their fears of him. Jay himself seems ready to leave.

Ann and I consent to a "trial run" before admitting Jay to the local service-system. He spends a weekend at a group home and at the sheltered workshop. There, and for reasons we cannot then explain, he attacks a housemate, Bernie. Bernie is a decade or so older than Jay, much more competent, verbal, friendly, and kind but also intellectually disabled. Bernie reassures us, "It's OK. I just call for help. I forgive Jay; he can't help it."

Cautious after the Bernie incidents but desperate, we accept the "slot" that has Jay's name on it, his entitlement to his adulthood. We cannot know just how much of a warning Jay has given us; our caution, though deserved, is far too modest. But we are ignorant at first how woeful our caution is.

The weekend comes for Jay to move out of our home. We invite friends and neighbors to a transition party. There is music, with Jay—in blazer, white shirt, and red tie—leading the singing. Our guests—adults and children alike—sing along; the children dance, putting on a show dedicated to Jay.

Friends speak to Jay and tell him how proud they are of him, how much they love him, and how happy they are for him.

There is laughter; there are tears of joy. Jay is launching into adulthood. He smiles broadly and laughs; he gives hugs and kisses to his friends. He is joyful, and blissfully ignorant.

Our friends have no idea what Jay is about to enter; we do, and we are hesitant, though hopeful. We do not reveal our feelings; this is the moment to celebrate Jay, not fear for him.

Choking

Jay's first week at the agency bodes ill for the future. He is in a group home, blandly called "the White House" because it sits on a lot adjacent to "the Gold House," each painted and named for their respective colors. Both are group homes, with about a half-dozen men in the White House and a similar number of women in the Gold House.

Jay begins his stay with a roommate and within a week is moved to a room by himself. He rebels, pulling pictures off the walls, tearing the mattress on his bed, and refusing to eat or get out of bed.

In the White House, one of Jay's housemates is an older, balding, taller, silent man, a star-gazer, lost in his own world. We do not know why but Jay simply cannot tolerate him.

Time and again, Jay tries to choke him. Staff pull him away from his victim and relocate him to another group home, across town. Jay continues to pursue his target, now in the sheltered workshop.

The man's mother is a state senator. We joke, after withdrawing Jay from the agency, that Jay understood self-determination better than any scientist: In choosing the son of a senator for his aggression, Jay assured his expulsion from the agency.

How smart he was! Or, if not that, how serendipitous was his behavior. It communicated to us as powerfully as any words could.

Bodyguards and Buddies

Jay is increasingly restricted. He is moved to a more restrictive home, one with more staff, fewer residents, and far away from the man he has choked. He is assigned to a "bodyguard" who physically restrains him whenever Jay become upset, which is to say, at least twice daily. Knowing no other way to behave, the staff resort to restraints and force to pull Jay out of bed, and water pistols, squirting water at him when he refuses to comply.

There is nothing private about Jay's behavior or the staff members' response to him. One day the "bodyguard" takes Jay to his barber for a haircut. Jay is agitated. The guard has been wrestling to pull Jay out of a car and then restrains him as he tries to flee. The barber, who is our friend, watches for a few minutes and then goes to Jay.

Jay stops struggling and becomes compliant. He sits in the barber's chair, peaceful. When the haircut is done, the "bodyguard" comes to get Jay. Jay resists, the guard struggles with him and finally forces him into the car.

Jay's barber calls Ann and me and tells us what has happened. "The next time I see anyone fighting with Jay, I'll punch him out. Jay's my friend. Is that OK?"

We caution against violence on Jay's behalf, but we are grateful that our friend cares enough about Jay to hold it in reserve for him. There are different kinds of bodyguards, and Jay knows the difference between those who do not truly care for him and those who do.

Jay is failing, and not for the first time. I recall the days, seventeen years earlier, when he refused to emit "aah" when put into a black room at the Kennedy Institute; bananas held no appeal for him then, and nothing that anyone can now do at the adult agency reduces his non-compliance.

In time, Ann and I understand that Jay was not the failure. The system was. Members of the system—the agency's employees—had an insufficient understanding of why Jay and others with disabilities are aggressive, depressed, and self-injurious. To the extent that any one understood applied behavior analysis, they failed to implement it with Jay, offering no rewards, only punishments; no choices, only coercion. Most of all, the agency's employees failed to recognize that Jay was rebelling against a system in which he had no choices about his life. The coercion to which he objected through his behaviors was not simply physical; it was profoundly psychological, too.

Kate's Question

Kate visits Jay at the group home. She is ten years old. She sees the grubby rugs, the sterile rooms, the bologna and sliced processed cheese and white Wonder Bread in the refrigerator, and the TV and VCR we gave the home, now broken. She notes how distant Jay is from the other people who live there, how the usual genuine friendships he had had in our home and neighborhood were utterly missing. Later that day, she questions us, "Why did you put Jay there? You wouldn't put me there. You wouldn't want to be there yourselves. Why is it alright for Jay to be there?"

How do we explain our choice? That we thought we had no choice but that program or nothing. The agency had a monopoly on services; we had come to the top of the waiting list and had to take "the slot" or be relegated to the bottom again. We were exhausted from advocating for him. We wanted time for her and Amy, and even for ourselves.

No explanations sufficed for our ten-year old, who understood and called us on the double standard. We had advocated for and preached equality but not been fully faithful; she saw the hypocrisy. We had failed her and Jay, and ourselves.

Quitting

Ann and I meet with the director and senior staff of the agency; they do not intend to do harm, but their system does not accommodate Jay, and they acknowledge as much. We then meet with the chairman of the board of directors and the agency's lawyer, a friend of ours. Ann serves on the board, attempting to secure reform from the inside. We offer to devote our time and talents to making the agency the best it can be. We aspire to excellence. We describe our vision.

The senior staff respond, "You are simply asking for an exception for your son. He can't do what you want him to do or be. You need to be realistic."

The chairman of the board adds his perspective, "We don't want to be excellent. We don't want to be out front or lagging behind. We just want to be in the middle."

Jay's aggression and self-injury continue, both at his group home and at work.

Seeking to know why Jay is failing at work and at group-home living, we ask him, "Where do you want to work?" He answers, "Wear a tie." We listen and understand: he wants to work where we work, in a place where there is a sense of dignity, not in a sheltered workshop. He points us toward a different way, but we do not immediately take that way. We err in accepting the "is" and not pursuing the "ought."

We ask Jay, "Where do you want to live?" He answers, "Sue and Dom." We understand: he wants to live in a home such as the one he had with Sue and Dom at Crystal Springs Nursery, in Massachusetts. Again he points us toward a different way, and again we err in too readily accepting "is" and not pursuing "ought."

We meet with the agency's director of vocational services—the man in charge of the sheltered workshop. We explain what we have tried to do and why we think Jay has behaved as he has. We express our frustration. He makes no offer to change any of Jay's circumstances. The agency has a one-size-fits-all model.

A few weeks later, we meet with two members of the agency's staff—both psychologists. We explain our hopes and expectations for Jay, and we express our deep frustrations that nothing has changed and is not likely to change for Jay or any other people served by the agency. Increasingly, our frustration becomes despair and despair becomes anger. One of the two psychologists says, "Good job, Ann, you are handling this all so well."

Ann responds, "No, I'm not, and don't tell me I am. Face it, this is all horrible for everyone, especially Jay."

Ann and I look at each other, and, a nano-second before we believe they are about to tell us that Jay must leave the system, we say, as if in unison, "We quit."

I speak, "We will fashion a life for Jay, the life he wants and deserves."

Ann adds, "This whole thing has not worked. We have to find our own way."

The other psychologist speaks, "What are you going to do when you fail?"

Ann is aghast, utterly speechless.

I rise, take Ann by the hand, and, leaving, respond angrily, "We aren't going to fail; we are going to succeed. And that's not a threat, that's a promise!"

Now, with no services for Jay at all, we bring him home, dragging him from our car and into our home, his depression such that he cannot or will not walk on his own.

On Our Own

That night, we lie in bed, his room next to ours, the girls downstairs in their own. We have no sense of where to go for help, what to do. But we recite Martin Luther King, Jr.'s phrase, "Free at last, free at last, thank God Almighty, we are free at last."

We determine to do Jay's life our own way, which is to say, his way, adhering to his choices to work where he can wear a tie and to live in a home such as Sue and Dom gave him. We decide that night to form a non-profit corporation. We call it, Full Citizenship. I create an acronym: FUCKYOU—Full Unadulterated Citizenship for Kids and Youth Opposed to Unemployment. FUCK YOU, we yell to the absent staff of the old service system. We are on a new road.

Now home with us, Jay has two affects. Sometimes, he is his usual, calm self; more often, he is depressed, sluggish, resistant, and glued to his bed.

We ask him, "What are you thinking, Jay? What do you want? Do you want to say anything to us?"

He answers, "Dirty, stinky, broken, busted, and throwed away."

Even until his last year of life, he would hear us speak the corporate name of the system and invoke his chant, "Dirty, stinky, broken, busted, and throwed away."

Blessed by a long-time memory and insistent on speaking or behaving his mind, Jay cannot be dissuaded from that chant. He had it right when he first spoke it. He had it right forever.

42

6

Integration in Bethesda

We take a sabbatical for fall, 1987 through summer, 1988. Funded by the Joseph P. Kennedy, Jr. Foundation to work in Washington, D. C., we are in a position to choose where to live in the metropolitan area. We ask our friends there, "Who is the best teacher you know, the best for Jay?" The answer is unanimous: Mary Morningstar. We learn where she will teach, and we locate in that school district, in Bethesda, Maryland.

It is about the second week after Jay has begun his last year in school, now at Walt Whitman High School. He will be twenty-one at the end of the school year and no longer eligible for a free appropriate public education. In many ways, we know this is a make-or-break year—his last chance at a formal education. We cannot, however, anticipate exactly how pivotal this year will be.

Mary is his teacher, trained at the University of Georgia and the University of Maryland. She is determined to secure Jay's effective education and authentic inclusion in a school that never before had had any students with significant disabilities.

"Cool"

We come to school to pick Jay up on a Friday afternoon. Mary walks with us to our car, uncharacteristically somber. Cautiously, she says, "I need to talk with you about something hard to mention."

We brace ourselves, for we think we have heard it all—about aggression, self-injury, touching other students, touching his genitals, and wetting. We are surprised, "Rud and Ann, I have to tell you, Jay is not wearing the right clothes."

We are relieved. It's just a matter of clothing.

She explains that the clothes Jay loves—the ones David Schwartzburg gave him, the white shoes and checked pants and bright shirts—are just "not cool." They make him stand out in all the wrong ways. She counsels, "Have your daughters go shopping with him tomorrow. They will know what he needs to wear." And so begins a friendship with Mary, and a technique of inclusion, that bodes well for Jay and us.

Imagery matters, especially when a person has a disability. And not just clothing-based imagery, but other as well. Mary knows that.

Not Unable

Mary arranges for Jay to accompany a student without a disability in picking up the attendance rosters from all classrooms during the first class period of each school day. The student and Jay do the job together for about two weeks. Then the student, with Mary's supervision, gradually steps aside to let Jay walk the corridors of a sprawling building, enter classrooms, pick up the rosters, and deliver them to the central office. In short order, it is time for Jay to do that work himself, by himself. He performs magnificently.

He does, however, make one major change from the previous routine. Rather than giving the rosters to a secretary, he takes them directly to the principal or assistant principal, bypassing the other administrative staff.

In his own way, he demonstrates to every student in every class every morning, and to each teacher and the administrators, that, though less able, he is still able.

The Letter Jacket

Mary is not content to have Jay be the attendance-roster collector. That is not sufficient high-status for him and her. She approaches the football coach, "Coach, I have the perfect student to be an assistant manager."

The coach accepts her offer.

Mary brings Jay to practice the next day, introduces him to the coach and his staff and to the manager, a pony-tailed co-ed. Mary does not know about Jay's hair-pulling, his fixation on pony-tails, and we do not tell her, fearing she will retreat from the integrating approaches she has used. Jay performs magnificently, giving towels to every player who comes off the field, whether the player needs a towel or not.

At the football banquet in December, Mary, Jay, Ann, and I sit alone, in the back of the banquet hall. We are still newcomers to Walt Whitman High School, not part of its "establishment."

The junior varsity team, coaches, and managers receive their letters.

Then the coach, seated on a platform with a member of Congress, the superintendent of Montgomery County schools, the principal and assistant principal, says, "Now for the varsity. I begin with the assistant manager, Jay Turnbull. Jay, come get your letter."

We are taken by surprise, but Jay, hearing his name, walks toward the platform. He arrives, standing below the coach. He has not observed, or, if he has observed, he has not heeded the custom of the night: The players stand below the platform, receiving their letters from the elevated coach. Jay tries to climb onto the platform and cannot. We are aghast. Football players rush toward him, boost him onto the stage, putting him where he wants to be but where he and other players have not belonged. The coach hands him his letter.

Parents and players have been silent. Now, they recognize him. "Oh, it's that boy, the one with the towels." They start to applaud. Their applause grows louder, and louder, and louder still. Jay pats himself on his back, obviously proud, joining the applause of the audience. The applause abates as Jay begins to leave the platform, sitting on its edge to fall to the floor. Players come to him, to help him down.

Now the applause crescendos again, louder than before, sustained as Jay walks to our table, his face in a broad smile.

Other managers and players receive their letters. The evening comes to a close, and we begin to leave.

Three women approach our table. We do not know them. They introduce themselves as the mothers of the tri-captains.

"Our sons want Jay to have a letter jacket. But, Jay's jacket will not arrive until May. He needs to have one now. So our boys drew lots to see which of them would give his letter jacket to Jay. On Monday, Jay will have his jacket. One of our boys will not, but all have given to Jay."

They leave, and we dissolve into tears. Towels and letter jackets, symbols of giving and receiving, emblems of inclusion. Jay wears his jacket through the summer; it is another layer of his skin.

He has become a full citizen.

A year ago to the day, we remember as we drive home, we had confronted the two psychologists in Lawrence and quit "the system."

Dance All Night

At the junior-senior prom, Jay brings a date, Jane Smith, the daughter of a good friend. Jane prefers to talk and eat with Jay's friends. Jay, however, insists on dancing each dance. Absent his date, he finds partners among the cheerleaders, pom-pom girls, and members of the school band—the young women who were part of the football enterprise, months earlier.

The school year comes to an end, seniors' yearbooks arrive, and students begin to autograph each others' books. Jay comes home with his yearbook, and we look for his picture inside. We find it, and then, as we close the book, we see the autographs on the inside front and rear covers, nearly a hundred of them.

They are testimonies to Jay. Young people, never before having gone to school with anyone with a disability, speak about Jay's meaning to them. He has transformed so many more people than football players, pom-pom girls, band-members, coaches, and administrators.

There is no going back to segregation. It is clear: we must continue to give Jay to his communities. To let him go, to turn him over, to have faith he will find his way among others and will elicit their goodness.

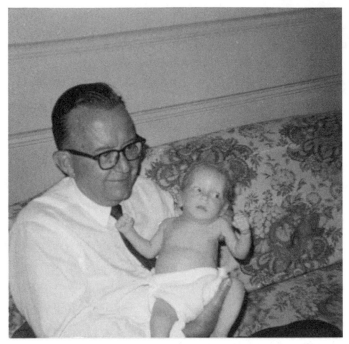

Jay, 3 months old, with my father, Henry Turnbull, 1967

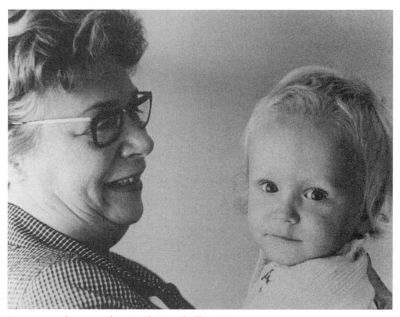

Jay, one, with my mother, Ruth Turnbull, 1968

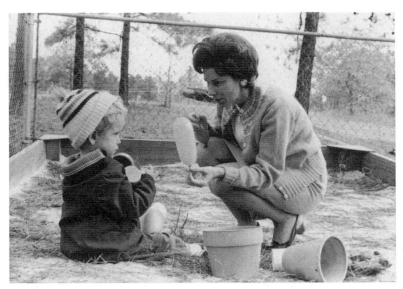

Jay, 3, with Evelyn Taylor, Sarah Barker Center, Durham, N.C., 1970

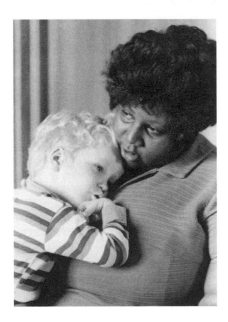

Jay, 3, with Cordelia Bethea, Sarah Barker Center, Durham, N.C., 1970

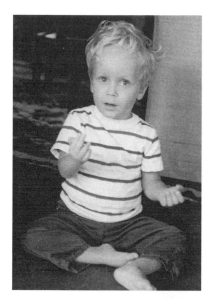

Jay, 3, Chapel Hill, N.C.

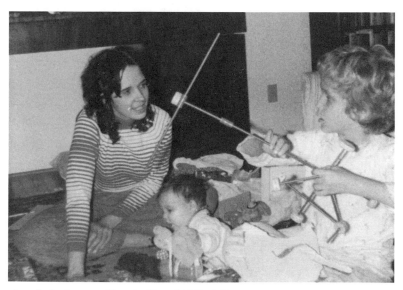

Ann, baby Amy, and Jay, 8, Chapel Hill, N.C., 1975

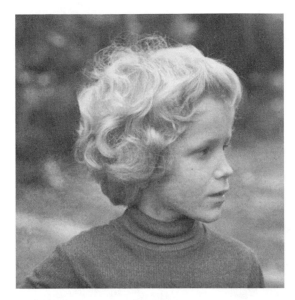

Jay, 8, Chapel Hill, N.C., 1975

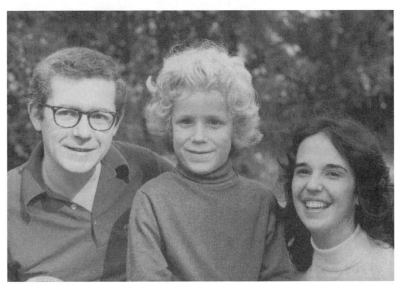

Jay, 8, with Ann and Rud, Chapel Hill, N.C., 1975

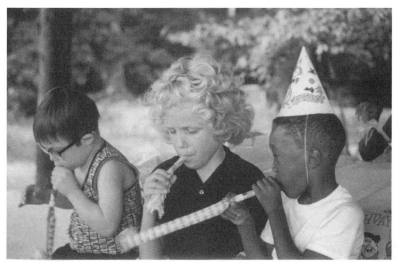

Jay, 8, with school-mates Bryan (left) and Christian (right), Chapel Hill, N.C., 1975

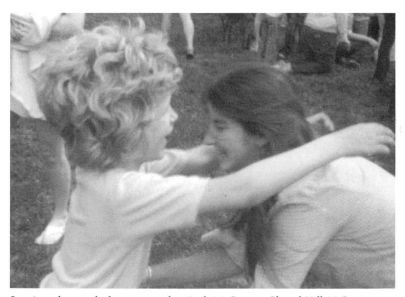

Jay, 8, with special education teacher Beth McGowan, Chapel Hill, N.C., 1975

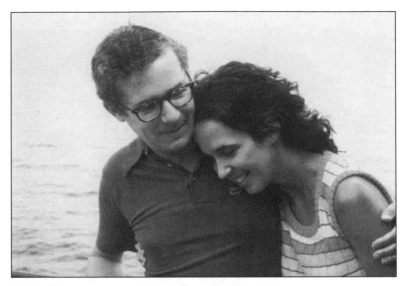

Rud and Ann, pregnant with Amy, Nantucket, Ma., 1974

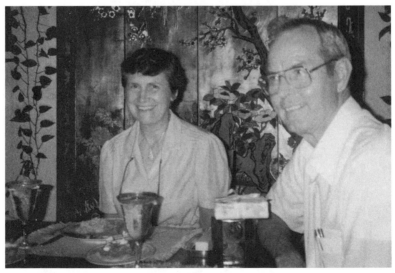

Dot and Jim Cansler, adoptive grandparents, Chapel Hill, N.C., 1976

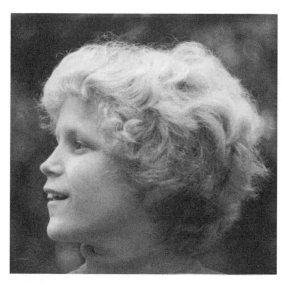

Jay, 9, Chapel Hill, N.C., 1976

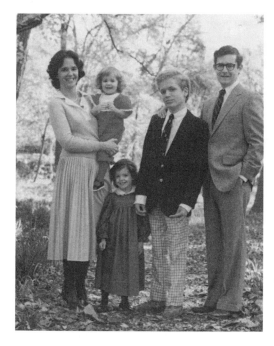

Ann, Kate (in Ann's arms), Amy, Jay, 12, and Rud, Chapel Hill, N.C., 1979

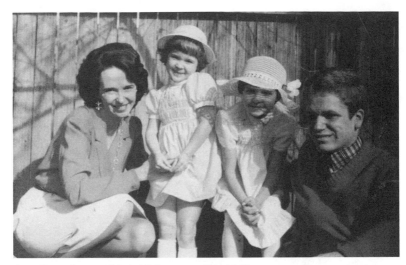

Ann, Kate, Amy, and Jay, 13, Lawrence, Ks., 1980

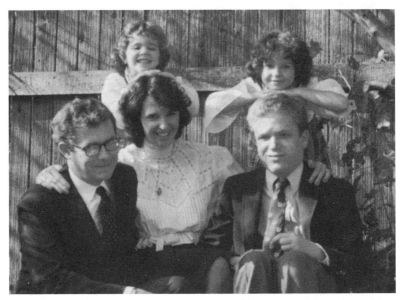

Kate and Amy (rear), with Rud, Ann, and Jay, 14, Lawrence, Ks., 1981

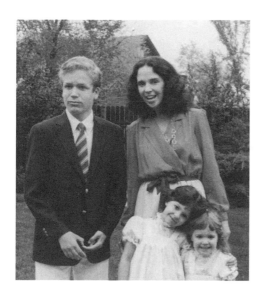

Jay, 15, Ann, Amy, and Kate,
Lawrence, Ks., 1982

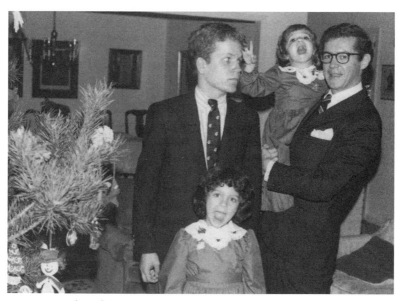

Jay, 16, Amy (front), Kate, and Rud, Lawrence, Ks., 1983

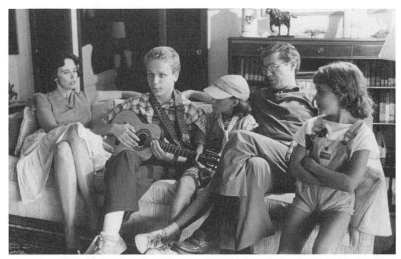

Ann, Jay, 18, Amy, Rud, and Kate, Lawrence, Ks.,1985

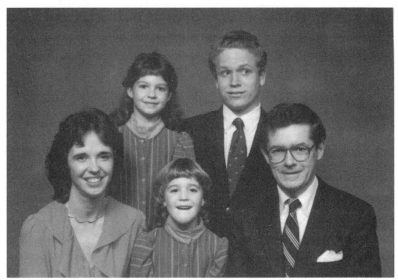

Amy and Jay, 20 (rear), Ann, Kate, and Rud (front), Lawrence, Ks., 1987

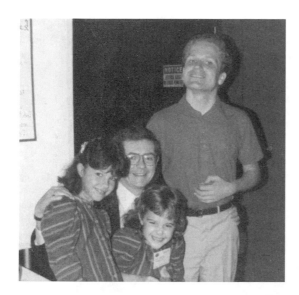

*Amy, Rud, Kate, and
Jay, 20, Philadelphia,
Pa., 1987*

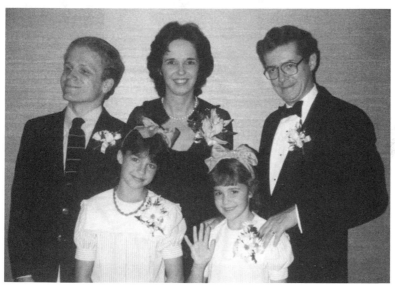

*Jay, 20, Ann, and Rud (rear), and Amy and Kate (front), Philadelphia, Pa.,
1987*

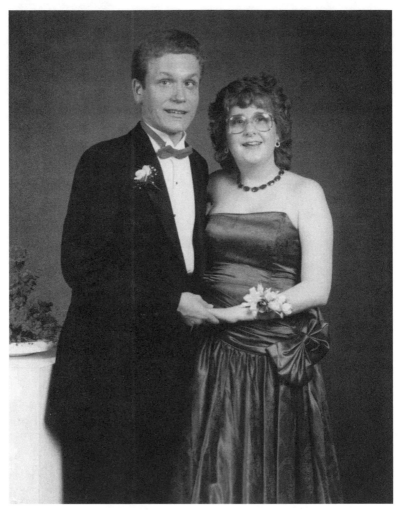

Jay, 21, with Jane Smith, senior prom, Walt Whitman High School, Bethesda, Md., 1988

PART II

The Man Himself

There is no truly logical place in this chronicle to describe Jay—the man himself, the disability categories into which he was classified, and his characteristics. Some of the essence of Jay and some of his characteristics—his charisma and natural ability to draw people to him and into his life, his sweetness, his love of music, his attractive demeanor—are apparent from the stories above. But by no means do those portray him fully.

To appreciate him in full, and the delights and challenges he brought to us and many others, it seems appropriate at this point in the chronicle to write as fully as possible about him. Having done so, I pick up the narrative about his life after Bethesda, the story of his enviable life—life in Lawrence, Kansas.

7

Jay's Classifications and Characteristics

Jay was born with hydrocephaly, a neurological condition that caused him to have intellectual disabilities (known as "mental retardation" or "mental deficiency" in those days). Later, he was classified as having autism and a rapid cycling bi-polar condition. During the episodes of aggression described below, he seemed to have seizures, but we were never able to persuade him to submit to an EEG examination and thus were unable to confirm or exclude classic petit or grand mal seizures.

Persistence and Anxiety

Jay is maddeningly persistent. When he wants us to do something, he asks, looks at us as if to be sure we understand, and then asks again. If we do not respond to what he wants, he repeats his routine, soon dropping the inquiring look and simply stating, over and again, his preferences. One story makes that point.

It is June, probably in 1991 but certainly not more than a year or two later. We celebrate his birthday at his home on Hilltop Drive.

(How he came to live in his own home is a story for later in this chronicle.) We expect just over a dozen friends. We have carefully arranged the food, drink, and knives, forks, plates, and napkins to be easily accessible; we have invited one of Jay's music therapists and she has brought her guitar. All is ready. Jay's first guests arrive. Jay looks at them, looks at us, and says, "Alvamar Drive," meaning he wants the party to move from his home to ours, on a street by that name.

We explain, "No, Jay, you have your home and your birthday party is here."

He demurs, not exactly calmly, "Alvamar Drive."

We try again, "Jay, we always have your birthday at your home."

More loudly and beginning to flap his hands and trot in place, he demands, "Alvamar Drive."

We see the explosion coming and assent, pack Jay and all the party gear into our car, leave a note for the unarrived guests, telling them where the party will reconvene, and go to Alvamar Drive.

Jay smiles broadly as we back out of his driveway and sings "Happy Birthday" to himself when we arrive at our home on Alvamar Drive.

The routine—ask, reject answer, ask again, reject answer, and ask and begin to tip over into an explosive episode—happens so often that we either yield or help him anticipate but not agitate about what will happen in his life. When it comes to important dates in the calendar year, we again accommodate.

That is because Jay is a walking calendar. He knows the common religious and secular holidays by name, something about their significance, and their sequence. His "year" begins with Christmas; then, in order, New Year's, Valentine's Day, Memorial Day, Fourth of July, Labor Day, Halloween, Thanksgiving, and Christmas again.

"Christmas soon," he implores.

"Yes, Jay, three weeks," for it is just after Thanksgiving.

"Soon," said impatiently.

"Yes, Jay, three weeks."

"When?" said anxiously.

"Three weeks. One, two, three."

"Three weeks?" now said urgently.

"Yes, Jay, three weeks. Let's count them. One, two, three."

He counts, and, daily thereafter, we tell him the number of weeks and days remaining. He counts with us. He softens. Anxiety leaves him. We sense it departing, for it is nearly palpable, concrete.

He anticipates these holidays; often, he seems to derive more pleasure from anticipating them than by participating in them. It is as though he wants them to be here and be gone, quickly. They disrupt his regular week.

True, the food is special and plentiful, and he enjoys that. He leads us in saying Grace, then gathers as many mashed potatoes and gravy—always a combination of brown and white gravy, per his command—onto a spoon, not the fork we have taught him to use, and ingests it in a single gulp. He smiles, eats heartily the rest of his meal, and then, anticipating dessert, repeats, "Pecan pie, Pecan pie, Pecan pie," the first phrase spoken in an even voice, the second with a lifted sing-song, and the third with a deep basso on the last word. He loves the eating part of holidays and, of course, the people and laughter; and, true too, he sleeps late and takes long naps. But these interludes interrupt his routine and his wedded-ness to it.

Body Language, OCD, and Predictability

Jay has limited communication skills; he can express his basic needs and preferences but complicated thoughts elude him. In compensation and as a short-cut to making his wishes known, he repetitiously uses his favorite phrases, but he also is an actor, though his "acting" is simply being himself. We learn to interpret his short-cuts, read his body language, and ensure as much predictability in his life as we can, thereby avoiding some of his more challenging behaviors.

A curled lip means he is angry. Tightened lips means he is anxious. When he puts his first finger and thumb together and wags his other three fingers, we know this calms him; it is as natural to him as breathing. But when he escalates this behavior, or begins to flap his hands in the air or clap them together, usually uncontrollably, we anticipate a behavioral outburst. At those moments, we try to smooth out his "high." We try to divert his attention to something pleasant. We take him to a room where he can have silence and a less stimulating environment or, if it comes to that, a place where he can erupt and we can prevent him from hurting himself.

He orders his world, arranging his immediate environment so that it pleases him, teaching us that we challenge him more than he challenges us.

Fans are to be inactive, never operating.

Each specific light switch must be either up or down, we cannot discover why one must be one way and another the other.

Closed doors in our offices—Ann's and mine—please him. He shuts them and us, mastering his immediate environment and proclaiming, as it were, that our research center is a place where he works and where his parents do not belong. This is his center, not ours; we belong at home, not here.

Post-it notes do not belong on doors, bulletin boards, walls, or, for that matter, anywhere at all.

Tables are meant to be walked around, especially the dining room table in our home, though the walk-around is the less direct route to his room from the dining room.

At his home, he always ascends to the second floor by way of the carpeted stairs and descends by way of the uncarpeted wood stairs.

He uses short and not un-curt phrases to signal what he wants: "Dad not spend the night" when I come to his home late in the afternoons.

The towel on the oven-door handle must always be pushed to the far right.

As soon as he finishes eating, usually before us, he takes his plate to the kitchen and returns to take ours away, ignoring that we are still eating.

When he believes a woman has overstayed her welcome, he searches for her purse and hands it to her. She has been "pursed." With men, it's the same: briefcases and back-packs handed to their owners means simply, "Goodbye."

He rehearses his daily routine, seeking the predictability and thereby becoming more adaptable and flexible when changes occur, as they invariably do.

He does not abide the living room chairs being other than flush against the walls.

TJ (the dog) must keep his "go-out-to-play" bell just at the corner of the back door of his home, never under the rug there.

Perseverance was built into him. He would repeat his requests over and over again until we yielded. If any piece of office or home equipment is broken, he repeats "It's broke, fix it now," and we try. If we fail to do so immediately, we try to buy time and respite from his constant reminders to fix that which is broken by promising "tomorrow" or "soon." "Soon" often does not work; it is too indefinite. So Jay responds to "soon" with "when." We offer a specific day. He is satisfied.

Communication

Like famous baseball announcers who coin and then repeat a phrase over and over again until it and the speaker become inseparable in the public's mind, so Jay has his own phrases.

"That's right"—he agrees with us.

"How does that sound?"—he is confirming his decision.

"Maybe later"—he procrastinates.

"I'm fine"—he politely refuses our request.

"Five minutes"—he begs off, ignoring a request.

"Pretty soon"—he delays, shilly-shallies.

We learn these phrases and their meaning only by responding in one way or another until Jay signals, by not repeating the phrase, that we have given the proper response. Others in Jay's life also learn what Jay means when he uses these phrases. Like us, they learn how to communicate with him and then how to enter his life, almost always on his terms and with delight that he and they are in sync with each other. Joy comes from that synchronization. We have learned to engage with Jay on his terms and thus taken huge strides in blunting some of his most challenging behaviors.

8
Challenging Behaviors

There is a radically different Jay than the one whose persistence demands attention. Few people outside our family and circle of close friends and care-givers know this Jay. This is the Jay of the hard times. Telling about him seems to dishonor him, to portray him in a most unfavorable light. Not to describe this Jay, however, is to falsify him and blunt the realities of his and our family's life. It is to minimize how truly gloriously he lived in spite of this other part of him, and how faithfully many people dedicated themselves so he would be the "real Jay," the man we described above and will describe even more, below, the man who lived an enviable life.

Aggression

Beginning in his late adolescence, Jay, whenever "wired" or upset, sometimes becomes spontaneously aggressive against us. When we sense his agitation, we do not often risk driving with him in the backseat of our car; he will often reach over to pull our hair. So we buckle him into the passenger seat in front. We also keep him a good distance away from Amy and Kate; they know not to come too close to him.

On trips into the community, he sometimes inexplicably becomes aggressive. At lunch with a colleague, he bolts out of the booth they share, runs across the room, and pulls the pony-tail of another diner. Accompanying a volunteer from our church to visit people from our church at a "retirement center," Jay pulls the hair of one of the cleaning staff.

It is not as if he never pulled people's hair before. When I would prepare to leave him after visiting in Rhode Island or Massachusetts, he would grab my hair and hold on to me fiercely. He would do the same whenever Ann, Amy, or Kate were with him and he was unsure whether they were preparing to leave him. When he had a solid purchase on our hair, he could keep us with him; he could prevent us from abandoning him, even if only temporarily.

We know better than to change his routine and at home we are on constant "watch" for Jay's behaviors. When he is wired or upset, and especially when he seems ready to erupt into aggression, Amy and Kate become hyper-cautious around him. The dynamic with their brother is changing, and not in ways we want.

We conclude that the more Jay senses we will leave him, the more he clings to us by grabbing our hair or wrapping his arms around our heads. We also conclude that the less choice Jay has, the worse his behaviors become. The more restricted he is, the more aggressive and non-compliant he becomes. The less positive behavior support there is, the less he responds with good behavior. Lack of choice leads to eruptions, depression, and resistance. Punishment leads to resistance.

Eruptions

Sometimes we can anticipate Jay's outbursts; other times, we cannot. When he signals an eruption that can lead to aggression, we know to remove him to a quiet place and try to contain him. But he does not always telegraph his behaviors. Each eruption nearly perfectly mirrors the preceding ones.

He becomes tighter and tighter, more and more wired. His eyes roll to the side of their sockets. He flaps his hands more and more uncontrollably and rapidly, speeding up his usual stereotypical hand-movements. He curls his lip up toward one ear or the other; he sticks out his lower lip; or he purses his lips or bites down on them. He begins to chant, usually saying "No, no" or, not speaking, making strange guttural or whooping noises. He begins to quiver, his legs seeming to have tremors. He stomps his feet, running in place. He begins to scratch his shoulders, back, groin, or legs. He digs at the cuticles of his fingernails, or puts his hands into his mouth, biting down on them but not breaking his skin.

He then enters a full-fledged outburst. He either runs in place or runs away, usually the former. He shrieks, a loud and repetitious "woo-woo." He flaps his hands vigorously, balls his fists and hits—or with an open hand slaps—his head or chest or, if he is sitting, his thighs. His face turns red; his heart beats powerfully and quickly. He usually cannot respond to our requests to "cool it" or "take a deep breath" or "put your hands up into the air."

If he is standing, we try to guide him to a couch or chair so he cannot run and so we can physically restrain him, holding his hands to his sides. If he is in public, we try to direct him to a car; he usually runs toward the car, seeking escape from whatever triggered his outburst.

As we restrain him, always asking him to "calm down" and reassuring him, "You are OK, Jay, relax," he will grab our eyeglasses, hair, or face. He will strike himself uncontrollably. When we try to protect him from himself, he hits us. If we hold his arms, he will try to hit his head against walls, floors, chairs and couches, or any nearby object, for we cannot restrain his hands and head at the same time.

We are careful to remove our eyeglasses and any pens or pencils or other sharp objects from our shirts and from anywhere within his reach.

These outbursts last for as few as two or three minutes or for as many as six to ten. Often, one outburst occurs, subsides, and then escalates into yet another, serially.

They end gradually, Jay becoming less and less agitated, not shrieking so much, not hurting himself so much. The de-escalations often begin as we restrain him and reassure him that he will be "OK." When they end, Jay is exhausted. Over and over again, he says, "I'm sorry."

He has exploded, his feelings have erupted, and now, like a volcano, he is dormant. He becomes silent, and he sleeps, usually for several hours. When he awakes, he is the "old" Jay, pleasant and not dangerous to himself or others.

Early on, we learn to detect the preludes—the mild tremor of the volcano, as it were—and we are sometimes able to forestall Jay's full outbursts by changing his immediate environment. We bring him to a quiet and low-lighted room; ask other people to leave the room where he is; turn down or off any radios, television, or CDs; sit beside him and hold his hand gently, using steady and low voices to reassure him that he will be alright. We ask him to lie down, rather than allow him to sit, or to sit, rather than stand, thereby minimizing his opportunity to flee from our supervision and support. If he is sitting on the floor, we try to move him to a chair or couch so he can not hit his head against the floor, as he does whenever he can during his outbursts. Sometimes, one of us—either Ann or I—tries to calm him down; sometimes, both of us try, but we learn Jay prefers to have only one person with him during these preludes.

As Jay's obsessive-compulsive behaviors increase—picking up paper from the floors of his office or public restrooms, turning lights on and off, removing "Post-it" or posted notices from doors and walls in the university buildings where he works—we go into a "red alert" mode, preparing for outbursts, making as regular and calm as possible Jay's environment, giving him as much choice as possible, including the choice to stay at home rather than go to work or to sit in a private room and on an easy chair at work rather than do his job at his desk.

Often, we succeed in thwarting an episode; sometimes, we fail. Jay's nature is such that, if he is bound to have an eruption, little can be done to prevent it. Inevitability becomes part of Jay's and our lives.

As scary as these episodes are, they never result in such injury to Jay or others that any medical treatment is necessary, and we never call 911 or take Jay to an emergency room. At their worst, the episodes result in bruising that persists for a few days, or in some torn skin tissue, usually the cuticles of his hands. Rarely are we ever injured; sometimes, Jay pulls our hair, but we hold his hand to our heads so he cannot pull, and in a few moments, he releases our hair and grabs at himself or at another part of our bodies, usually our torsos.

When Amy, Kate, and Jay live with us, Amy, even as a young child, tries to take control; she commands, "Stop it, Jay! Calm down, Jay!"

She is too young and too small to become physically engaged and stays arms' length away from him, calling for us to come to her aid. Sometimes she cannot stay out of his grasp; he is quicker when in these states. He bruises her. When they inquire about a bruise, she explains to her friends, "I bumped into a door last night while going to the bathroom."

Kate flees to Margaret Ann Schwartzburg's home, next door, but never says why. Simultaneously, she protects both herself and him.

Ann and I acknowledge a frightful fact: There was a form of domestic violence in our home—the fear of violence and, sometimes, its very presence.

In our first home in Lawrence, we move the girls to two bedrooms downstairs and Jay to a bedroom next to ours, trying to create a safety-zone, a no-man's land where fear is absent. In Bethesda and then in our second house in Lawrence, we do likewise. Jay's behavior shapes the type of house we buy—its layout must accommodate to his actions.

We learn what we have to do for Jay and ourselves during these episodes, and we tell his roommates and daytime care-givers what the preludes are and how to protect Jay and themselves during the behaviors.

We prepare little notices, plasticize them, and put them into Jay's wallet. They tell anyone who reads them who Jay is, where he lives and works, how to contact us or his roommates, what to do and what not to do, and that Jay has a disability and does not engage in these episodes intentionally, that they are involuntary responses to stresses or conditions he finds objectionable.

Depression

Depression is the obverse of aggression and eruptions. Jay becomes lethargic; it is as though a powerful fatigue grips him. He moves slowly, falls asleep at work or elsewhere, remains in his bed for a day or so, not eating or drinking, pulling the covers up to his chin and grabbing them tight whenever we approach to try to coax him out of bed. During his most severe depressions, Jay remains in bed for three or four days, rising only (and infrequently) to go to the toilet. He disrupts his medication regimen.

When we offer food or liquid, he shuts his mouth tightly and pulls the covers over his head. When we try to massage his jaws to get him to open them, he pushes us away.

Sometimes he will go to the kitchen table and eat only a few foods; ice cream or soda pop appeal to him. These infrequent meals (such as they are) give us the chance to crush his meds, mix them into the ice cream or put them into his drink, and continue the medication regimen his doctors have prescribed. Without these deceptions, Jay would have no medication.

Often, he refuses to respond to his roommates; in desperation, they call us, and we go to him, sometimes being successful in persuading him to rise out of bed or leave his safety-chair behind. Sometimes, persuasion fails, and we become drill sergeants, barking out orders, trying to take control of Jay's psyche. Sometimes, we succeed; more often, we fail and are obliged to wait out Jay's depressions. We learn they will end; we learn the worst part of each episode does not last for more than three or four days, usually two or three.

We know Jay does not want to be depressed, that he dislikes these times as much as we do, but he cannot will himself to be his usual cheerful self. His biology controls his behaviors, and all the various medications we have administered, under physicians' orders, do not block the depression; they only make the depression less frequent and less severe.

Documenting "That Jay"

The most challenging episodes of aggression, eruption, and depression began when Jay was in his middle-teen years. They persisted until he died. And they became part of the public record. That is so because Jay began to receive Medicaid-funded Home and Community Based Services when he was eighteen and because, to qualify for services, we had to describe fully Jay's aggression, eruption, and depression.

To qualify Jay for services, we annually meet with a social worker from the local developmental disabilities agency and complete a form that determines the nature and extent of Jay's disability, his behaviors, and his needs. We pay particular attention to the questions concerning his behaviors. We are careful to read the definitions of each of the "qualifying" behaviors before answering the questions. When we do not know whether to describe Jay as more or less able/disabled, we chose disability. The state has made Mafioso of us all.

We state the number of times during the past year that Jay has engaged in any of the following behaviors:

hav014ing tantrums or emotional outbursts

damaging own or others' property

assaulting others physically

disrupting others' activities

being verbally or gesturally abusive

engaging in self-injury

teasing or harassing peers

resisting supervision

running or wandering away

stealing

eating inedible objects

displaying sexually inappropriate behavior

smearing feces

Compulsorily, we give information about his physical, psychiatric, and dental examinations. We list the medically prescribed interventions necessary to prevent his physical and behavioral challenges and the names of the people who provide speech therapy, massage therapy, yoga therapy, and music therapy. We describe the residential and employment support he receives and the names of the people who provide the support.

We describe his fine and gross motor skills, his functional literacy, his ability to understand and respond to requests and to communicate, his self-care skills, and his independent living skills (or lack of skills), such as making his bed, cleaning his room, doing laundry, using a telephone, shopping for a simple meal, preparing food that does not require cooking, using a stove or microwave, crossing the street in a residential neighborhood, using public transportation, and managing his own money.

We point out that Jay has a behavior intervention plan written and supervised by specialists in positive behavior support; must live in a carefully structured environment to avoid or mitigate behavior problems; must be restrained physically or guided away from individuals or settings that cause him to act out; and requires one-on-one supervision for many program activities.

We identify Amy McCart and Laura Riffel, specialists in behavior support, as the key members of Jay's behavior-intervention team. They have studied with us in their doctoral programs and know both Jay and us. They have designed a data-collection system that will satisfy the demands for evidence of Jay's behavior. We describe the system in detail.

The system requires everyone who has daily contact with Jay to record data on Jay's behaviors at four segments of each day—while he is preparing for work, while he is working, while he is not working in the afternoons, and during the time between dinner and bedtime. The system also requires scoring on a scale of 0 to 5, indicating whether Jay has a little or great amount of aggression, obsessive compulsive disorder (OCD), or depression. Finally, it prescribes the interventions that Jay's care-givers, co-workers, and family will use if he is aggressive or either too obsessive or too depressed.

To be certain that we can prove Jay's eligibility, each of us involved with Jay also collect data on a form that matches the state's criteria for eligibility for services and levels of support and funding. If Jay engages in a "score-able" behavior, we note it on both forms—

ours and the state's. Now we have two sets of comparable evidence to prove Jay's eligibility. By recording the behavior that earns him "points" that qualify him for funding, we fixate on his challenges.

I attach a memorandum to the annual report about Jay, with an attached diagram, explaining the relationship of the therapies to Jay's behavior and behavior states; a copy of his positive behavior support plan; and a copy of his typical weekly schedule. I note that we track thirteen different behaviors, of which only eleven are included on the state's form.

I then list eleven different therapies Jay receives, the professionals who provide the services and the two data-collection systems we use daily to chart his behaviors and remind his care-givers how to intervene, and I state that the particular therapies are effective. I attach the illustration of the relationship of the therapies to his behaviors, including those that the state deems to trigger a higher score on the annual assessment. I update this report annually for 2007 and 2008. We have no need of it for 2009; Jay has died.

This approach is perverse, for, every time he scores a point, we recognize that we have failed to intervene sufficiently. He does not want to be a point-getter; we do not want him to challenge us; and we certainly do not want to have weekly and often daily reminders that the behaviors he started during his adolescence have persisted into his adulthood.

It is not enough for the state that we must elaborately detail Jay's behaviors and needs and how we respond to them. The state also requires us to complete annually yet another form, the Life-Care Plan. This plan requires us to re-state Jay's behaviors and his needs. But it also requires us to develop a budget detailing how we will use the Medicaid funds to which Jay is entitled.

The budget identifies Jay's residential support team, the independent contractors who will provide various services (internal medicine, dentistry, psychiatry, music therapy, speech therapy, yoga and massage therapy, etc.), the nature of Jay's participation in the community (what he will do each day), the costs of medicines, the amount of the deductibles his insurance programs leave to us to pay, costs of travel to physicians, and the costs of background checks, high-speed internet connections, accountant services, workman's compensation, and public liability insurance. Increasingly, Jay's budget reflects that there is a business model underlying Jay's support.

As much as Ann and I understand that we must collect data, describe Jay's behaviors (only the difficult ones, not the charming ones), and his disabilities (only those, not his abilities), we find ourselves in the position of having to describe Jay only partially, not to portray the real Jay. He is not the person of the documents; he is far more.

Reliable Allies

So many years, so many forms, so much data—it is impossible for Ann and me to do it all alone. Nor do we try. We enlist "reliable allies." They include his many annually rotating job-coaches—people who taught him how to work more effectively and independently. Among them were four who came to his funeral—Dorothy Johanning, Richard Viloria, Jane Gnojek, and Lauren Priest. There were others, each loyal to Jay, each respectful of his strengths and needs.

Also joining Jay's circle of support were his housemates, Jesus and Shala Rosales, Tom Allison, Elizabeth Giffin, Lilly Cusick, Anne Guthrie and Richard Gaeta, and Tom and Laura Riffel and their sons Bryan and Brandon.

Still other people entered the circle—music therapists, speech-language therapists, members of fraternities who participated in the

Natural Ties program that Jay, Pat Hughes, and Corey Royer started in 1990, and our friends and colleagues.

So many people, so many forms, so much data—yet such candid conversation and deep devotion to Jay and each other. Co-workers, Ann, and I are Jay's "regulars." We talk, send emails, write daily into a notebook that Jay carries with him everywhere he goes, meet on a regular basis and enlist young people, his "irregulars," to support Jay and thus us.

To understand just how many people are needed to support Jay, add to the members of his circle of support the physicians who see him for regular checkups and for various diagnostic and surgical procedures, his psychiatrist, various psychologists, his yoga instructor, his massage therapist, and—most of all—Amy and Kate, his sisters.

An Intentional Family

We are creating more than a circle of support. More than that, we are creating an intentional family. As the many people who support Jay communicate with each other, they develop personal bonds; Jay is the mortar binding one person to another. Each person becomes an agent for Jay, an advocate for him, and then, in turn, an advocate for each other.

There is a notion that a circle of support consists of people surrounding a person with a disability. In Jay's life, however, the circle consists of people surrounding each other, not just Jay, to support each other wherever and whenever Jay enters our lives and even beyond the Jay-focused aspects of our lives.

Jay brings us together in common cause, but the common cause is not just Jay alone; it is also each other.

No Silver Bullet

We do more than create an intentional family and rely on the talents each person brings. We seek advice and treatment from professionals whom we know or are recommended by other professionals whom we trust. We learn that no one person has all of the answers, much less as many as might begin to help, and that there is more than one desirable approach to supporting Jay, blunting the aggression, eruptions, and depression, and bringing joy to his life. There is no silver bullet, no perfect single answer.

Colleagues at the University of North Carolina at Chapel Hill evaluate Jay when he is sixteen and in semi-catatonic depression. They are specialists in autism, conclude he has autism, and recommend behavioral interventions. We have tried them; we try again. We are too often unsuccessful.

Jay continues to be almost chronically depressed and frequently aggressive. We take him to a for a week's in-patient evaluation at an out-of-state psychiatric institute, where yet other colleagues work.

We receive still another evaluation—but the same diagnosis: intellectual disability and autism. We do receive, however, a somewhat different recommendation: group home living and behavior modification—predictably, "gentle teaching," a form of more positive, less punishing behavior modification. We reject the first recommendation and try the second. Again, it makes little difference. It could be that Jay and the intervention are not a good match, or it could be that we are inept in using it and engaging others to use it. Whatever the cause, we continue to misread Jay and to fail to pin down exactly what will purge his aggression, eruptions, and depression and restore him to his usual sweet self.

We turn to other usual places for help. First, to Menninger's, in Topeka, and then to the department of psychiatry at Kansas University Medical Center. Physicians at both places recommend the then-standard regimen of medication. Jay continues to be depressed and sometimes aggressive.

Upon the recommendation of old and close friends, we hire a psychiatrist on the staff at the medical school in Chapel Hill. He spends two days with us and Jay and recommends a new drug, Tegretol. Jay begins a lifetime regimen of Tegretol, together with semi-annual blood-draws to monitor its effect on his liver.

Soon thereafter, we hire two behavioral psychologists to evaluate Jay. They spend three days with him and leave us with a complete report, more than a dozen pages of data, analyses, findings, and recommendations. Both have understood Jay and his environment; both have confirmed causes that we suspected and both have made suggestions we implement.

Jay begins to have fewer challenges, but we correctly foresee that his aggression and eruptions are simply part of him, an inherent aspect that we will have to minimize but live with for the rest of our lives with him. There is only so much of a person's biology and psyche we can change, and only so much of a person's environment we can control.

Wet

Jay's aggression—like his depression—is accompanied by his frequent bed-wetting. We hire a post-doctoral fellow at the University of Kansas, a man whom we knew in Chapel Hill when he was a student there. Early every morning, he comes to our home, often before 6 a.m., sometimes even in the middle of the night, and begins the "dry day" routine: get Jay out of bed, go to the bathroom, and shower.

The man's devotion to Jay is obvious; his skills in reinforcing Jay to get out of bed and go to the bathroom just as soon as he wakes up are impressive; his diligence in performing his work never flags; and our efforts to assist him are reliable. Yet, there is something about Jay that not even this highly trained and committed psychologist could remediate permanently, though his work was far more effective than we ever had hoped and persisted for the rest of Jay's life. But wetness is just part of Jay—an occasional part, but still part. Jay will continue to wet his bed at least weekly for the rest of his life.

Chaos and the Barometer

We consult our colleagues at the university who specialize in human development, applied behavior analysis, and communication and social skills. We also turn to Doug Guess, a colleague in our department who has carried out research on the bio-behavioral states of children with significant disabilities—the children who rotate between alertness and withdrawal. He proffers the chaos theory— the world sometimes seems chaotic to Jay, so he responds chaotically, sometimes dangerously, and sometimes childishly, by wetting his bed. We change our charting scheme to try to capture the chaotic, poltergeist-like stimuli and Jay's responses.

Laura Riffel, Jay's job coach for two years and later his housemate, studies Jay carefully each day. She, like us, acknowledges Jay is uncomfortable when rains come. "Stop raining soon?" he asks. And asks again and again. He is more anxious when it snows. "No more snow!" he demands. He fears walking in it. When the sidewalks are clear and there is no snow, he pulls away from us if we want to take his hand or arm to support him as he walks down stairs or crosses a street. When the snow is on the ground, he leans heavily on us. Rain and snow make him edgy. Laura hypothesizes, "Jay's moods are linked to the barometer." If so, and it is a plausible theory, what can we do? Chaos and the weather are beyond our control. At times, Jay is, too.

Reconstructing "Challenging Behaviors"

Our professional friends widely regard Jay's behavior, and the comparable behavior of others with disabilities, as "challenging." That is so because they challenge those of us who are professionals or family members.

He is at his best, his true self, when only his intellectual disability affects him. Then, he is social, happy, a man with the mind of a child. Jay's hard times are not caused by his intellectual disability, but by the combination of autism and bi-polar disorder. Both, of course, are constant factors in his life. But sometimes they are dormant, allowing his intellectual disability to exist by itself.

At other times, they are active and seem to supersede his intellectual disability. At those times, he experiences the withdrawal and obsessions and compulsions of autism, and the intermittent self-injurious behavior, aggression, and depression of his bi-polar condition. These manifestations, coupled with his inability to express his needs and choices other than by behavior, are the roots of his challenges.

They mask and disguise the authentic Jay, too often blocking his ability to give and receive the love he wants and that others want to give him. Jay hates his autism and bi-polarity. He knows they do not reflect his true self. Others know it too, and their knowledge gives them the ability to accept and love him as he is.

Over time, we recognize a deficiency in the professional construct that Jay or others with disabilities "emit challenging behaviors." It is not so much that Jay's behaviors challenge us as that our lack of understanding of Jay and failure to respond to his choices challenge him.

We are the challengers; Jay is the challenged. The more we change, the less he challenges.

We also realize, to our great regret as professionals, that so many professionals, and the systems within which they were trained and worked, are unable to help Jay and us, as much as we need their help and as much as they want to help. His education in Chapel Hill consisted of enthusiastic and dedicated teachers. His education in Lawrence was less than adequate, limited because of his teachers' low expectations and inadequate abilities. His education in Bethesda was superb simply because of one teacher, Mary Morningstar, and the good hearts of so many students, faculty, and staff.

With a few exceptions, the physicians, psychologists, music therapists, and speech-language therapists who worked for Jay with us were exceptionally able professionals, committed to Jay and us but, despite their best efforts, not sufficiently integrated with each other. The professional and financing systems within which they worked did not support integrated service.

The adult service system in Lawrence was not at all acceptable to Jay or us. When we left it, we were on our own, and that, in the long run, was best for Jay and us. Yet the amount of time we had to devote to creating a life of dignity for Jay was enormous and incalculable. It was not only us—his parents and sisters—who had to construct that life for Jay. Over the twenty years of his life, beginning when we left the traditional system until he died, there were approximately 300 individuals involved in supporting him with our guidance.

Few parents or other family members can do for their children what we did for Jay. That is the tragic conclusion we reach. After all the years of creating and implementing rights and all the public and private funds spent to create a service system, it comes down to parents and brothers and sisters themselves.

We turn the world upside down, focusing not on Jay but on ourselves, reversing our perspectives about Jay and ourselves. We first look at ourselves, and then at Jay. We learn to change ourselves, and in doing so to change Jay's behaviors. It is, after all, his life first and foremost, and ours next.

We also acknowledge that none of the genuinely competent professionals and others supporting Jay wanted only to change Jay. Instead, they wanted to create a good life for him by accepting him as he was and then building on that essence. They sought the real, inner, authentic Jay, and he responded. Their ability nurtured his abilities; their compassion spurred his competence; their devotion parented his development; and their love for him begat his for them.

9

Therapies for Wellness and Integration

Jay sometimes has these challenging behaviors. At other times, he is simply delightful. What makes the difference? Bit by bit, we learn that there is no one answer.

Music: The Key

When I heard Jay speak his first words, when he was at Pine Harbor Nursery, he sang "Michael, Row Your Boat Ashore." After Ann and I brought him home to live with us, he was still without words unless he was singing—with my mother, it was "Bye Bye Blackbird," and with Ann's father, it was "You get a line, I'll get a pole, and we'll go down to the crawdad hole." Music literally rang his chimes. It was the entry-point into his spirit, the vehicle for his joy. Desperate for a way to combat Jay's depression, we turn to Jay's love of music.

We call Alice Ann Darrow, a professor of music therapy, and ask, "Would you help us bring some joy into Jay's life by connecting him with your students? He loves music."

She meets him and agrees. Within a week, she tells us she has found a music therapy student to work him. He is Sterling McNay, a Canadian bassoonist. He spends a year with Jay, teaching him the rudiments of how to hold and strum a guitar.

Della Clayton succeeds him, and, in succession, nearly fifty other students, at least one each semester, sometimes more, enter his life. Some work a semester and leave. Others, like Gayla Berry, stay with him year after year. Two of them, Elizabeth Giffin and Lillie Cusick, become his housemates. Music fills his home; Jay dances and sings, sometimes solo, sometimes in duet. We have found a way to add great joy to Jay's life and, not incidentally, to forestall his outbursts and depression.

The Jay-T Shuffle

Della forms a band, Black Cat Bone. She plays keyboard and sings, accompanied by a guitarist and bassist, drummer, and trumpeter. She invites Jay to The Jazzhaus, a local music-and-dance venue, to hear the band. The Jazzhaus is on the second floor of a downtown building. It is old, smells of stale beer. Its bathrooms are ancient, the bar multicolored with neon advertising.

His housemate drives him to the bar, and Jay enters unaccompanied, for Della awaits him. He enters sits at a table that Della reserved for him. The place is packed; Della is locally famous, a "rocker." It is midnight. Jay is wired.

She begins a set. Jay goes to the dance floor and dances. He places his feet firmly on the floor, pointed way outward, evidencing his splay-footed, hip-displacement. He does not move them, but he swings his hips left to right and back again, raising his arms over his head. He dances alone. The nearly 100 other patrons, drinking and smoking, stare at him. They don't know him. None rises to dance. Jay is soloing.

Della completes the set and announces, "OK, guys, you have just seen the latest dance craze in Lawrence, the 'JT Shuffle.' Let's all join Jay and shuffle with him."

She reprises the set, and Jay, never having left the dance floor, now sweating profusely, starts to dance again.

A few couples join him; more come to the floor. Soon, the dance floor is jammed, everyone dancing the JT Shuffle.

Now, JT no longer dances alone and is no longer different. Everyone does his dance.

They join him in his ways.

In time, we all join him in his ways. The less able among us lead us all.

The Beatles and Mouthwash

Jay favors The Beatles. His choice is significant because their music becomes a tool for changing his behavior.

Jay dislikes mouthwash and cannot prevent himself from entering our bathrooms and pouring it out.

His music therapist, Mike Brownell, learns we are upset about this behavior and have failed to dissuade Jay from being wasteful. We see Jay's perseveration as a problem, as evidence of an obsessive-compulsive condition. We are correct, and we are more than a bit peeved.

Mike devises a solution. He teaches Jay modified lyrics to one of the Beatles' songs, "Let It Be."

> *When I find myself in mother's bathroom,*
> *And I see the mouthwash standing there,*
> *I know I must not touch it,*
> *Let it be, let it be.*

The Brownell solution works. We adopt it and, with other music therapists, adapt other songs. We find the key, we turn it, and Jay changes.

Music and a Bad Place

Gayla Berry is one of his Monday night regular music therapists. She nearly always brings Dana Gates, one of Jay's classmates from his days in special education in Lawrence, to Jay's for dinner and music.

Their routine begins with "Hello, JT," a song that includes, one after the other, at least a dozen of Jay's friends and family members. Jay and Dana finish singing it; Dana is the last person he names in the song. Then he turns to her and says, "Dana, I love you, I love you."

Gayla interrupts, "No way, José."

Jay laughs, and Dana says, "I love you, José."

Jay laughs again.

Dana sits next to Jay on a couch; she has a castanet, tambourine, or rattle in one hand, and pounds Jay's knee and thigh with the other, unable to control her movements. "Be careful," says Gayla, "you don't want to hurt Jay in a bad place."

Neither Jay nor Dana understands. To protect Jay, Gayla asks them to move apart.

Speech Therapy

Relying on the good will of another colleague, Jane Wegner, the director of the university's speech-language-hearing clinic, we secure the services of graduate students in that program to work with Jay for an hour or two each week. That work begins in the mid 1990s. It entails lessons on how to communicate with others—not how to enunciate a word but how to be a partner in the give-and-take of conversation. Jay learns. When he is "up" or engaged, he is a good conversationalist. When he is depressed or eruptive, there is no semblance of conversation. But speech therapy entails more than being a conversationalist.

Safety Drills

Kansas experiences tornados, and prudence dictates that Jay should know to go to the basement of his house if the tornado siren sounds. Under Jane's weekly guidance, students from the speech-language clinic make picture books of a tornado and record the sounds of a tornado siren. Weekly, they rehearse the sounds and teach Jay to retreat to his basement. Safety is the value-added of speech therapy.

Telephone Manners

Jane and the students also teach Jay how to dial "911"—a huge safety issue—and how to ask and answer questions and politely tell the person on the line that he has finished talking with them. These are lessons about communication, though the medium is the telephone and telephone manners.

Jay has learned too well his lessons from the speech-language therapists about talking on the telephone. Tom receives a call, Jay reaches for the telephone. Tom holds the telephone, Jay reaches again. Now Tom walks away from Jay. Jay follows him. Tom cannot escape. He surrenders the phone to Jay, who says "Hello," "How are you?", or "Goodbye," depending on what he wants from the person holding the phone in his presence. He has learned his manners, just not all of them.

Bobby is on the cell phone, talking to Tom. Jay wants to talk to him so badly that he picks up the cordless phone, "Hello, Tom, hello." No answer. Jay hangs up and goes to find Bobby, not fooled for long.

"My name is…."

To assist Jay to engage in conversations, Jane and the students ask Jay how he wants to be addressed. Jay's given name is Jesse, for my ex-wife's father, and Lawrence, for a Turnbull-family scion. We never use those names. Instead, we use the names he wants. He prefers "Jay" and "JT" and insists we and others use those names for him. He names himself, giving himself his own identity.

To me, however, he is Mr. T., Mr. Turnbull, Buddy, Buddy Man, Main Man, Hey Big Guy, Big Ticket, Jaaaay-T-T- T-man, Son, and Old Boy (which always prompts him to correct me: "Old MAN"). He responds to all. Between us, naming is a flexible matter.

Bad Words

One of the consequences of Jay's deep presence in our community and among young people, and of his frequent watching of television, is that he hears words he should not use. We are careful to teach him not to use those words, but we do not always succeed.

It is Christmas-time at the Schwartzburgs', sometime in the mid-1990s. Katie and Laurie Schwartzburg are there; our daughters Amy and Kate are, too. There is glee everywhere, music played and sung by Schwartzburg cousins, bright decorations and a scrumptious dinner by Margaret Ann, liquor poured freely by David. Jay delights in the sights, sounds, smells, the embraces from the women, the handshakes from the men.

Margaret Ann's friends arrive from St. Louis. They are wealthy, sophisticated, and well-dressed. Jay intrudes into a conversation they are having with Ann and me. He turns to Ann and says, "Don't touch your penis in public."

The guests are aghast. They had not known what to make of Jay and now he confounds them even more. Ann is caught unawares, uncharacteristically silent. And then Jay adds, "And don't talk about touching your penis in public."

Ann turns to the sophisticates, "Jay has such good manners!"

We have learned to adapt, to cover for him.

Alternative Health and Wellness

Also at about the same time we arrange for Jay to become involved with music and therapy programs, we secure weekly therapeutic massage and, separately, weekly yoga for him. These are our wellness approaches, the means for forestalling his challenging behaviors, eruptions, and depressions. They yield benefits. Jay's physical health remains robust—he rarely has a cold or flu. And his emotional health improves—he is less frequently "wired."

Together with music and speech therapy, these increase the number of people he associates with each week, the variety of activities he has each week, and his choices—he now has a choice to be engaged or to simply stay at home, sleeping or watching television.

We find that these therapies—music, speech, and alternative wellness approaches—reduce the frequency and intensity of Jay's outbursts and depression. But we acknowledge that we have limited ability to support Jay during the times when outbursts and depression occur. We resign ourselves to the inevitable: Jay has these outbursts and depressions; they are his inherent characteristics, just as other characteristics are inherent.

Reluctantly and over time, we grudgingly welcome the outburst-depression characteristics. They force us to admit our own limitations, to try harder to understand the world from Jay's perspective, to "become" Jay as it were, to stand in his shoes. We then begin to shape his world in such a way that it eliminates, to the maximum extent possible, the unpredictability, instability, lack of choices, and lack of engagement .

We discern the activities he likes and add them to his life; we identify the kinds of people he enjoys, and we bring them into his circle of support; we prepare him for holidays and bad weather, and tell him that the holidays will end (whereupon he tells us about the next one) and that the snow/sleet/ice/rain will be gone soon, even tomorrow, as he insists.

Choice, engagement, variety of people and activities, predictability, stability, positive behavior supports, and medication constitute our responses to Jay. As we increase each, except medication, which we stabilize, Jay succumbs to fewer and fewer rages and has fewer and fewer depressions. Jay chose the life he wanted. When he had it, he was joyful, delightful. When he did not, he was withdrawn, non-compliant, self-injurious, and aggressive.

10
The Joy Quotient

Jay's IQ ranges from the low to mid-40s. His adaptive behavior has not been scored according to any of the standard assessments, but we know that it varies depending on the presence or absence of his emotional-behavioral challenges.

We do not discount any of the efforts Jay's co-workers, job coaches, behavioral specialists, housemates, and friends make to increase his capacities. Indeed, we value them greatly and initially fret when we sense that Jay has hit a plateau and that those in his circle are content to maintain him there, rather than teach him new skills.

In time, however, we learn that a plateau is more like a ceiling. It seems that Jay has learned as much as he needs to know to live happily in Lawrence and work effectively at the university, and he knows that. He is comfortable with himself. When he wants to be independent, he is. When he wants help, he asks for it; and when he needs help, friends, professionals and family, including Amy and Kate, while they are living in Lawrence, provide it.

We come to understand that, as important as Jay's IQ (cognitive skills) and adaptive behaviors are, they are less important than Jay's

"JQ"—his joy quotient.

There is a correlation between IQ and adaptive behavior, on the one hand, and the joy quotient on the other. The higher Jay's joy quotient, the higher his functioning intellectually and behaviorally. Likewise, the more joy he has in life, the greater his intellectual and behavioral skills.

We acknowledge no difference between Jay and ourselves: the more we enjoy our lives and the duties attendant to them, the more competent we are, and vice-versa.

Jay teaches the value of the JQ and its relationship to the standard measures of capacity and functioning. Sadly, many professionals do not know his lesson; there are no validated measures of joy.

Jay, then, combines excesses in both joy and competence as well as in challenges—his rages, his retreat into his cocoon of depression, nearly catatonic sometimes, his biological shut-downs. Just as we are about to give up on him, to yield to our anger or despair, he becomes the Jay he wants to be, becoming beloved.

Tom Allison wrote us after Jay died, "Just as Jay was about to push you over the edge, he broke our hearts and won them back again."

11
The Intimacy of Care-Giving

Jay is competent in so many ways and incompetent in so many others. His competence lies in making known what he wants by asking or acting to secure the outcomes he wants. His incompetence lies in some aspects of caring for himself. From the very first days Jay is with us, Ann and I learn that we must support Jay to be a gentleman.

That means we must teach him manners and assure that he is as presentable as possible at all times. He likes being "Gentleman Jay"— the phrase we use when talking with him about how he grooms and dresses, and he describes himself that way when we are assisting him in his grooming and dressing. He would not be the gentleman he is without a significant amount of support from Ann and me and then from his roommates, Anne Guthrie and Richard Gaeta, and Laura, Tom, Bryan, and Brandon Riffel and the other members of his circle of support. There are many care-givers, all loving and considerate of him, all according him dignity in the most intimate of care-giving.

Our Physicality

I am one of those care-givers, telling him to wash his penis and "clean your crack," usually adding my touch to his imperfect bathing. With me and only me, Jay does not have a shy reaction—the recoil when someone touches his genitals. He allows me to use the washcloth on him. Other care-givers must use a long-handle brush. These are intimate cleanings, reserved for father and son, as though he were not a grown man but still an infant. He trusts me. When I am away from home, Ann's physicality with Jay mirrors mine.

We were truly of one body, and not just in the seminal sense. These father-and-son rituals were our bonds of touch—wash and shave routine in the shower; dry him everywhere; de-wax his ears after the shower or in the office between visits to our home; cut his fingernails; help him pull on socks; untie and retie his knotted shoes; button his shirt; tuck it in; make sure he has his wallet and keys; put on his watch—he held it out to me, always interrupting my dressing, always asking for everything to be in place and same order.

Through giving him such varieties of care for forty-one years, I had become part of him, even as he, upon receiving my love and giving me his, had become part of me, not only in the biological way but also in the daily ways of ordinary life.

Binding Acts

There were so many other little daily acts that bound Jay, Ann, and me in the daily ways of our ordinary lives—exchanging his special handshake (borrowed from his time with the SAE fraternity and improved upon by his brother-in-law, Rahul); rubbing noses ("nosey, nosey," he would say, tilting his head up toward me); inserting his belt into every loop on his pants; adjusting his socks to fit properly on his feet; unknotting his shoe laces and retying his shoes for him; reminding him not to ball up the paper towels but to dry his hands with them and then ball them up; cautioning him to use his soft "church voice" at church and elsewhere if he was too loud; buttoning his coat against the winter wind; asking him to walk more quickly or to put his feet down, left and right, left and right, as he descended stairs; begging him not to "roll" before passing gas, not to remove signs on the doors at work, not to pick up paper towels on the floors of public restrooms; imploring him to brush his teeth, top and bottom, front and back; rousing him from sleep when he could not stay awake at work, to get out of the easy chair in our conference room and "be a man and go to work." Together with Ann, I care for this man-child, our son, in ways that create and confirm an intimacy of love and trust.

Jay's World, Not Ours

With others, Ann and I try to modify Jay's behavior. But he modifies ours, requiring us and others to relate to him in ways he prescribes. Through his autism, he makes us all a bit autistic. We enter his world and, together, we live in the new "our" world, the one Jay creates.

Ann, Amy, Kate, he, I play games with each other, our own games. Sometimes, we play them as a duet—Jay and one of us; sometimes, ensemble, Jay and more than one of us. We reveal our family when we infrequently play them in others' company. Usually, these are our games—strictly within the family.

We grab each other's knees, squeeze, and say, "Gilly Wally got your corn." Or we tap each other on the knee; or grab each other gently by the nose or ear; or rub our noses together; or play "Hunga Hunga." I put a blanket over my head, spread my arms like a rooster, and approach Jay, swaying and saying "Hunga Hunga" in a low gravelly voice, always emitting laughter from him, always covering him with the blanket (of love), and always being told, "More." Amy, Kate, and Ann imitate me, eliciting the same delight from Jay.

In the elevators at home or work, I put my baseball hat on backward or bill-to-the-side, and Jay reaches to fit it properly, bill-front. I feint backwards; he reaches, grabs the hat, and triumphs as I square-up in front of him. He smiles. He knows he has won. And then I restart the game immediately. I give him every victory I can devise. He has earned them, simply by being who he is and pushing us as he does.

The list goes on and on. There was not a day when he, Ann, Amy, Kate, Jay, and I were in the same town together when he and at least one of us did not interact in some way or another; we were utterly Siamese. These were easy acts, not solely because they were for our son and thus done lovingly, but also because they were natural, as natural to us as our own acts are to ourselves.

Each of us becomes nearly the man Jay is: a grown man with an IQ of a six-year-old boy, the behaviors of a clown, and the delight of a child. Jay converts us to his world. He transforms. And not, of course, in just this way.

Incorporation

He was so much "with" me in so many small ways—those trivial, taken-for-granted ways that cumulatively made him such an intrinsic part of me.

Amy and Kate are part of me, though not in the same way Jay was. Amy and Kate, each in her own way, connect to my essence—not just biologically but also in habits of heart and mind and in essence of soul. Their physical dependence is, however, a matter long past, and I write here of fleshly, daily, taken-for-granted acts—acts of father-son incorporation: the action of making a single person out of two.

Jay and I were incorporated into each other in the physical, fleshly ways that come from forty-one and a half years of love and caring, of each of us doing the loving and knowing of the love of the other, knowing what it means to be loved.

PART III

A Life of Dignity

12
Paying His Way

For Jay to be a full citizen and all he wants to be—and all we want him to be—it is not enough that he has a home of his own and a safety net below him. He must be engaged during the day, for engagement blunts his difficult behaviors. More than that, work brings income, enlarges his self-esteem, and demonstrates to all that he can contribute and be productive. Behavioral, economic, psychological, and policy imperatives drive Jay and us in one direction only: Jay must work.

Hired, Fired, and Hired Again

Before we take our sabbatical in Washington and move to Bethesda in 1987, Jay receives job-training services from the state vocational rehabilitation agency. The agency provides funds so we can hire a job coach, someone who will teach Jay how to perform a job, with support, for at least twenty hours a week, at no less than the minimum wage, in an integrated setting.

We advertise the job coaching position and hire Nancy Hickham, whose willingness to work with Jay and lively personality over-ride her lack of experience with people with disabilities. Jay and she work at the main branch of the Kansas University library. His job is to put magnetic strips into books and thus make them relatively theft-proof. At the end of the six months' training period, the library staff dismiss Jay. He has failed at his first job, not for lack of commitment by Nancy but because he does not have systematic training in how to do the job. The books arrive and must quickly be theft-proofed and made available to the library's customers. It is not just about Jay or Nancy, but about the job demands.

There were no reasonable accommodations and, even if there had been, not a sufficient attitude or skills on the part of Jay's co-workers, other than Nancy, to make them. But Nancy is loyal and cheerful, and Jay likes her. When we move to Bethesda, we ask Nancy to come with us as our live-in aide, helping us take care of Jay, Amy, and Kate. She accepts and we go to Bethesda.

We return to Lawrence in the summer of 1988. Jay is now twenty-two, no longer eligible to attend school and only recently prepared, by Mary Morningstar at Walt Whitman High School, to hold a real job, one where he can wear a tie if he wants to.

Making Work Happen

A former doctoral student of Ann's and mine, Jean Ann Summers, now directs a federally funded project. She has served on the board of directors of Full Citizenship, Inc. and hires Jay. A few months later, Jay moves from her payroll to ours, for we have just received a five-year federal grant to operate a research center on family support.

The university's nepotism rules pose a challenge. We may not hire, supervise, or evaluate a member of our family. We read the rules carefully; they are structured in either/or language, allowing us to hire and supervise Jay but not to evaluate him.

Our new grant, however, is formally and legally awarded to an umbrella research entity. Its director, Dick Schiefelbusch, recruited us to KU. Its finance director, Ed Zamarripa, earned his doctorate under our mentorship.

They confer and announce, "It's easy. Ed will evaluate Jay. Put him to work."

And so it is that Jay begins the first of almost twenty-one full years' service to KU, working at the Beach Center and contributing to its work and the general mission of the university's magnificent disability programs: to advance the quality of life of individuals and families affected by disability through research, teaching, and service.

We have earned our way at KU; we have won Dick and Ed's respect and loyalty. Dick retires. Our friend from Chapel Hill, Steve Schroeder, is his successor—the same Steve Schroeder who gave Jay a pipe, the same one who is married to Carolyn, Jay's early psychologist. In time, Steve retires, and Steve Warren takes his place. He sees every reason to continue the evaluation arrangement: Jay is a good worker. But he is not thoroughly independent.

Support at Work

Jay needs support to retrieve the mail from and deliver it to offices in three different buildings; learn his way inside these large buildings; operate a postage machine and a duplicating machine; pick up paper for recycling, shred it, bag it, and put it out for collectors; clean our break room and refrigerator and coffee pot; clean bulletin and black/white boards; do university errands off campus; serve food when we are hosting lunches in our conference room; and help tidy up after the lunches are over.

He learned some of these skills under Mary Morningstar's tutelage at Walt Whitman High School, but he needs permanent support. Our federal grants allow us to hire him and a job coach who doubles as an office assistant. Over the twenty years when Jay works at the Beach Center, he has nearly twenty job coaches. One of them, Laura Riffel, becomes a doctoral student under our advisement, one of the two specialists who develop Jay's positive behavior support plan, and, in time, becomes Jay's housemate. Another, Lauren Priest, also enters the graduate program under our advisement. Others take different jobs and more responsibility at the Center or elsewhere at the university. Their launching pad is as Jay's coach.

Graduate students working with us are fascinated by him. Many offer to take him to lunch off campus or to eat in the break room with him. None is a more loyal lunch partner than are Richard Viloria, Karrie Shogren, and Nina Zuna. No staff person is more faithful than are Lois Weldon and Jane Gnojek. Lois is our administrative assistant; she knows nearly everything about us and unfailingly supported us to support Jay ever since she joined our staff in 1994. Jane is our fiscal affairs officer and joined around the year 2000. Students from the U.S. and from Korea and China become his friends. Jiyeon Park and Suk Hyung Lee, from Korea, become his gentle colleagues, bringing their soft and calm selves into his life, being constantly calming influences. He delights many colleagues and is delighted by them.

The Central Event: Testimony from Colleagues

Personal loyalty and nepotism have opened the door for Jay. But Jay has kept it open by being an effective worker and gregarious colleague. Nearly daily he proves his economic worth, and he wins people's hearts. The proof of his winsomeness comes twice in the late fall of 2009, some ten months after Jay dies.

At the annual meeting of the researchers at the Life Span Institute, the new director, John Colombo, details the Institute's financial growth and its researchers' honors. He looks at Ann and me and says:

"But the central event of this year was not about any of us or our success in competing for research grants. It was that our friend and colleague Jay Turnbull died."

We are stunned. Our colleagues respectfully remain silent for a minute, paying tribute to Jay, their colleague, our son.

Teaching How to be a Friend

At work, Jay daily takes the mail from the Beach Center to another unit, in another building. There, his friend Steve Schroeder waves at Jay, but Jay passes him by and goes to the next office down the hall. It is Ed Zamarripa's. Jay interrupts Ed at work, insists on his special handshake, tells Ed, "Open the door." Ed welcomes Jay and delights in Jay's affection and routinization of Ed's day.

When Ed is in a conference meeting, Jay ignores the many researchers gathered around, enters the conference room, reaches over the scientists to give Ed his daily handshake, and leaves. Jay teaches the researchers that personal conduct is essential and that modifying it or, worse, eliminating it, is not a legitimate object of their science of behavior modification. He teaches, instead, about community and affection.

Their routine—the open door, the insistently offered and happily received handshake, no matter the business at hand—is invariable. And it offers a lesson.

When Ed's colleagues convene to honor him upon his retirement after forty years' service, Jay has already died. The director of the Life Span Institute lauds Ed; previous directors praise him. Ed responds, thanking them and identifying the members of his family who are there and expressing his gratitude for their support.

Then, in the company of nearly 200 researchers and support staff with whom he has worked, he thanks Ann for teaching him about family quality of life and me for teaching him about public policy.

Now he pauses, visibly emotional, his voice cracks, and he says, "And I must thank Jay Turnbull, who taught me to be a friend."

Ed turns to us, nods, and sits down. Jay lies in his grave, honored.

We knew Jay had transformative power; we just did not know how deeply personal it was for our friends and colleagues.

13
The Enviable Life

When Jay is in his late thirties, Ann speaks to a large gathering of families and professionals, tells about Jay and his life, and characterizes it as "an enviable life." By using the term "enviable," she recalls the conversation she, Kate, and I had with each other after Kate had visited Jay in his group home and challenged us about the double standard we accepted: one kind of life for us, and another, far less dignifying one for Jay.

Kate has asked us to face up to the fact that, by admitting Jay to the community service system, we have asked him to settle for a life that we would not want for ourselves. We understood her challenge to ask us, "Why don't you have a life for Jay that you would want for yourselves, one you would envy if you were Jay?"

Ann and I debate whether "enviable" is the term we want to use. I say that "envy" denotes a sinful mind. She counters that "envy" sets a high bar for families and parents to achieve and characterizes an ideal. I yield.

From that moment on, we talk about Jay's life as "enviable" and explain the meaning we ascribe to that word—a meaning that conveys joy. The more we write and speak about Jay and his life, the more we realize that his is indeed an enviable life, not just in the way he lives it and in the way we shape it, but also in the sense that he inspires other families and professionals to seek a comparable life for people who have significant needs for support.

To tell about his enviable life, we must begin where we ended Chapter 6, "Integration in Bethesda."

Seeking Full Citizenship

Our sabbaticals completed, we leave Bethesda in 1988, determined to recruit Mary Morningstar, Jay's teacher, to be a doctoral student with whom we would work, intent to replicate the experiences at Walt Whitman High School, and utterly at a loss on how to achieve these great expectations.

We return to Lawrence and Full Citizenship, Inc., the corporation we formed when we quit the local service system. We have hand-selected our board of directors: parents of Jay's peers with disabilities, two professors of human development, the university's general counsel, and a local disability activist.

We now use the corporation for Jay's and others' benefit; running it is our second job, one that demands as much time as our university jobs. We make time for Jay and Full Citizenship, adding our duties to it to our obligations to our work and to Amy and Kate. We do not calculate the amount of time we devote to Jay, Amy, Kate, our jobs, and the corporation. We simply have our priorities—full citizenship for Jay, the enviable life; equally full and joyful lives for our daughters; and full discharge of our professional duties. It is not easy to balance these claims. Indeed, at times it is exhausting and nearly overwhelming.

We go to allies in the state's vocational rehabilitation agency, our caps in our hands, "handicapped" in the original sense of the word, seeking funds to operate the agency.

We secure funding to hire an executive director. We surround her with our doctoral students. Soon, Mary Morningstar, whom we have succeeded in recruiting to be our doctoral student, becomes the executive director.

She and others secure a grant, its purpose being to help Jay and others get jobs outside of workshops. Supported employment has begun, and we want Jay to experience it. The initial grant expires after two years, but other funding follows. We are less handicapped than before; we have some control over our destiny, some ability to shape Jay's life as he wants it, to work where he can wear a tie.

Slight autonomy derives from slight resources.

The Fraternity

Also on our return to Lawrence from Bethesda, we hire Chuck Rhodes, a graduate student in human development, to spend one afternoon each week with Jay. Our colleagues Jim Sherman and Jan Sheldon have recommended him to us; he is a graduate student in their program in applied behavior analysis.

Chuck's once-a-week routine consists of taking Jay to the SAE fraternity house, where Chuck is the resident advisor. Jay hangs out there. We tell our friend, the vice chancellor for student affairs, about Jay's new funhouse. He is visibly shocked and tells us that SAE has been on probation more than any other fraternity. We disregard Dave's implicit warning to avoid that fraternity. Jay likes Chuck, and no harm seems imminent.

Jay meets Pat Hughes, who becomes Jay's fraternity big brother. Pat calls late one night. "Rud, the chapter members have voted to make Jay a member. Is that OK with you?" I answer, "Yes." Ann concurs. One of our dreams is coming true: Jay has a place to be with young men his own age, an alternative to the segregated world he has rejected.

I don't add that my fantasy is for Jay to be initiated into a sorority, though that nearly happens when Kate Schwartzburg (our next door neighbor) and her sorority sisters in Pi Kappa Phi become his companions, some for pay, some for free as they carry out their sorority's community service obligation.

It does not matter to Jay whether the young people who are becoming part of his life are hired or not. What matters is that he has friends, they accept him, they engage him in wholesome activities, and he delights in them. Nor does it matter much to us whether the young people are employed by us, earn academic credit by having Jay as a "practicum" experience, or are with him simply out of friendship. What matters is that Jay is engaged with people who are devoted to him and that he obviously enjoys them.

Jay eats at the fraternity house every Wednesday night; sometimes, he attends parties there, often on Father's Day or Mother's Day.

Jay fits. Jay is changing—he is engaged with people his own age and is happy to be with them. There is nothing he does—picking his nose, passing gas, or scratching his genitals—that they do not do. He can make any bodily noises he wants, scratch whenever and wherever he itches, sleep in public, or dance wildly to the music. Whatever he would be expelled from a group home for doing, he does freely at the fraternity house. What constitutes unacceptable behavior in some circles is absolutely normal in others. Normalcy is a matter of place and people.

Natural Ties

Pat Hughes believes he has been called to the disability field, that Jay beckoned him to serve. So Pat establishes a college program that links students with adults with disabilities. He calls it "Natural Ties." The tie—the connection between the student and the adult—is natural, but it must be supervised, and I become the faculty advisor to the group. Jay is the catalyst for it; Pat and Corey are the initial leaders. Later, Jay affiliates with Kappa Sigma, where T. J. Trum and Andy Whitehead become his buddies. Many students enter Jay's life.

One of the popular movies of the time is *Rainman,* about a man (played by Tom Cruise) whose brother (Dustin Hoffman) has lived in an institution. Cruise removes Hoffman from the institution, begins to accept him as a man with autism who also is a mathematics savant, and becomes his friend and advocate, more than the absent brother he had been. Pat and Corey become the Tom Cruise character. Jay is "Rainman." Life imitates art. So what if it is Hollywood? The means are comparatively irrelevant when weighed against the result.

14
Three Young Men

Pat and Corey have now known Jay for two years. They telephone us one day and say they have a plan for themselves. It involves Jay. It is that they and Jay will live together in an apartment or house in Lawrence, beginning in the summer after they graduate. Ann and I consider carefully what it will mean for us, for Amy and Kate, for Pat and Corey, and, most of all, for Jay. We recall his days in the group home and now believe that it is time to try again to have Jay be more independent of us. Jay has failed at congregate care living and wants his independence from Ann, me, Amy, and Kate.

Truth be told, we also want to have our own lives, closely connected to Jay but more on our terms than his. His terms control when he is with us. We seek to balance the claims our daughters are making with the claims that Jay is making—and believe that we can do that better if Jay lives on his own, with all the support from us and others he needs. Thus begins Jay's life apart from his family, yet not apart from us at all. With Pat, Corey, and Jay, we scout out apartments and condominiums, visit them, and decide they simply will not do. We turn instead to the residential-home market.

Life Apart

Our neighbor David Schwartzburg tells of a house a friend is offering to sell. We look at it. We want to buy. But we need money. We call the trustee of a trust that my ex-wife's family had created for Jay. We explain what Jay needs, what we need, and what his sisters, now in their adolescence, also need. The trustee, for whom I had worked when first admitted to practice law in Maryland, agrees to buy a half-interest in the house if we buy the other half-interest. He tells us, "This is the only time the bank (a co-trustee that I represented when practicing) has owned property outside of Maryland."

Great expectations now align with significant resources.

With the trust's assistance and with a mortgage from a bank in Lawrence, Ann and I buy a modest one-story slab-house in an old, established neighborhood. Jay's bedroom and bath are on the south side; a large living room centers the house and leads to a kitchen on the east and a porch on the west; two bedrooms and bath are on the north. The living room becomes the common room—Jay and his housemates have little choice but to retreat or be together.

Pat and Corey live with Jay on a rent-free, utility-free basis. In exchange for basically free living accommodations, they contribute their time during weekdays to support Jay—a "sweat equity" arrangement. Jay comes to our home on weekends, giving them respite and, more importantly, giving us family time with him.

There will be more togetherness than retreat—sometimes, too much togetherness. We cannot foresee that yet; all we see is opportunity. Two young men—Pat and Corey—have shown us a path we had seen but feared to travel: Jay, living on his own.

Not in My Backyard

It is moving day in August, 1990. Pat and Corey are unloading Jay's and their furniture from a van. They are shirtless and energetic. They set up a "boom box" on the front steps; it broadcasts popular music to them as they work, and to neighbors, too.

A neighbor walks across the street, from his home to Jay's. He introduces himself again; we had met before. "I have to say, Rud and Ann, that I have some deep concerns about what you are doing."

I brace myself: here it comes, the NIMBY—Not In My Back Yard—prejudice against a person with a disability. "Tell me," I respond. "It is best to be candid."

Ann and I nod our heads, signifying we will understand his concerns, prompting him to tell us everything on his mind, and all the while preparing our responses. "Well," he replies, "It's not Jay whom I worry about. He's a gentleman. It's those two fraternity boys. What will the neighborhood become with them living here?"

We are visibly relieved. We explain our plans to supervise and promise to respond to any concerns he or other neighbors have. He and we agree: we will work this out, for Jay's sake.

I call Pat and Corey to meet us. "Guys, put your shirts on and don't go outside without them. Keep the noise down. And be sure to invite Jay's neighbors to a cook-out next week. You have to act like men now. Yes, you are in college but here, you have to be men."

Jay now elevates others' status. By living with them, he vouches for them, making them more acceptable.

Deviance juxtaposition is a concept in the disability world. It refers to the practice of placing people with disabilities in institutions near people who have been convicted of a crime and imprisoned.

In Lawrence, deviance juxtaposition takes on a new meaning: a person with a disability living with fraternity men. And NIMBY also acquires a new meaning: No Fraternity Boys In My Back Yard. Jay is exempt from NIMBY-ism.

Routines and Road Trips

For a few months, Jay flourishes with Pat and Corey. They are lively, energetic, and undemanding. With Jay's needs and preferences always in mind, they and we try to establish a regular routine—when to start the day, what to do regularly each day, when to close the day. It is not easy to comply with the routine. Simply because they are enrolled at the university, still active in their fraternity, and have families and a social life of their own, predictability is elusive. The more elusive it is, the more Jay challenges them and us by shutting down or resisting. One story illustrates how spontaneity or change of routine conflict with Jay's need for predictability.

Pat, Corey, and Jay undertake a road trip, Lawrence to Wisconsin, to attend a conference to tell about Jay's life and their roles in it. En route, Jay explodes. They continue their trip, restraining Jay to protect him and themselves. They keep the trip short, returning Jay, now exhausted from acting out and not sleeping well in a strange bed, to our home. We do not want to blame them for not turning back; they are young, ill-trained, well-intentioned, and bound for a family reunion. Instead, we blame ourselves: Have we put Jay in harm's way by entrusting him to them? Have we put them in harm's way? How do we extricate Jay and ourselves from an unacceptable situation?

To Jay, their world—and thus his—is chaotic. He needs predictability. So, predictably, his challenging behaviors return: aggression, self-injurious behavior, depression, and refusal to get out of bed. They misconceive what Jay will enjoy, never expecting to upset him, always wanting to include them in their up-beat life.

Pat and Corey leave after a year. They have they set us on two paths, for which we have been always grateful. They regarded Jay as capable of living on his own and they pushed us to give him what he had wanted but could not have asked for except by his behaviors—a home of his own. And they connected him to undergraduates through the program built around Jay, "Natural Ties."

15

Housemates

So much of Jay's enviable life and his participation in his community depend on how other people choose to support him. They can regard his behaviors as challenging, or regard themselves as his challengers. They can offer him work and value him and his contributions. They can commit several years of their lives to living with him. But the "they" changes. People come and go in Jay's life. That is problematic given Jay's need for stability and predictability. The question for us is how we can assure stability and predictability while also assuring that Jay will live on his own, as he wants, and participate as a full citizen in his community—how can he have the enviable life. We find answers in remarkable individuals—those who chose to live with Jay, to be part of the Turnbulls' intentional family.

Jesus and Shahla: Fundamental Interventions

When Pat and Corey notify us they are leaving, we must replace them. There is no prospect that Jay will leave his home and return to ours on an indefinite basis. Again with the help of our colleagues Jim Sherman and Jan Sheldon, we find new housemates. They are married and are graduate students in human development—Jesus and Shahla Rosales. They become Jay's housemates. Soon Corey, who has lived in Australia for a year, returns and becomes another housemate.

Jesus and Shala are older than Corey and are students earning their doctorates in applied behavior analysis. Corey, too, enrolls in graduate study in the same discipline. Together, they use the techniques of applied behavior analysis to create a more predictable world for Jay.

They counsel against medication and favor using only applied behavior analysis approaches. For a while, we concur, but they and we learn, in short order, that Jay needs the drugs that psychiatrists have prescribed. We now are firmly and irrevocably committed to mixed interventions, with change of Jay's environment being the fundamental intervention.

In time, Jesus and Shahla earn their degrees and leave, but they help us find successors. We now have few responsibilities in recruiting them; the roommates select their successors, knowing Jay and the recruits, fitting each to the other. Each becomes like a family member to Jay, finding their ways into his and our hearts.

The Feeder System

Building a community around Jay—an intentional family, a community, not a formal system of paid, professional services—takes work. The work is harder at the beginning. There is the business of asking close friends to recommend people and putting "the word" out through our networks; we do not resort to advertising. There is the business of interviewing, of taking the measure of the person's character, competence, and commitment; and of disclosing Jay's nature, his good and endearing traits as well as his challenging behaviors and how we respond to his needs.

In time, the selection business closes. It is no longer necessary for us to recruit and screen Jay's potential housemates. His present housemates and those who are in Jay's network recruit and vouch for the "recruits." Jay, like a major league professional athletic team, has his own feeder system. We, rather much like absentee owners, become involved only at the point of a final decision. We still want to interview, but since the recruiters—those who have been with Jay and are now leaving him—have selected the recruits only after having had them become deeply involved with Jay, our meeting with the new people is more a formality than a necessity of care-giving. Jay benefits from a process of natural selection.

Anne Guthrie and Richard Gaeta:
Four Years of Hospitality and Stability

We have accepted Anne Guthrie into our doctoral program. She is the daughter of Bob Guthrie, the scientist who discovered the PKU (phenylketonuria) condition and a powerful means for preventing disability in newborns; Anne is also the sister of Tom Guthrie, a man with an intellectual disability.

Anne's partner is Richard Gaeta, a New Yorker through and through, a creative painter, a marvelous chef, and a man with a heart as warm as Italy in summer.

They learn that Jay is about to experience yet another turn-over in roommates and, over barbeque dinner at their rented home in Lawrence one summer night, ask to be Jay's housemates. Knowing Bob Guthrie as well as we do, and having come to know Anne through her studies with us and Richard as a bon vivant, and anticipating that Anne will be with us for at least another three years, we accept.

They move in, and now Jay begins to settle into his adult years. He is in his late twenties, his adolescent biological changes well behind him, his medication regularized, and his behavior plan relatively well implemented.

Anne and Richard are inviters, collecting friends from throughout the community and hosting parties, delighting Jay and enlarging his circle of friends.

Richard hires on as a chef at the Mercantile Cooperative Exchange and soon Jay is a volunteer there, helping clear tables and pick up trash. He is beginning to have a life rather much like anyone else's—work for pay, and participation in his community as a volunteer.

Nonetheless, Jay has not been "cured" of his challenging behavior. Not at all. He still has behavioral outbursts; when frustrated, he sometimes breaks Richard's eyeglasses; he still refuses to rise from bed some mornings.

Anne and Richard leave after four years of living with Jay. They have added extraordinary zest to his life by simply being themselves and inviting so many people whom they know into their and Jay's home. They have faced and overcome Jay's behavioral challenges. They set out for Washington state, where Anne has family and professional prospects.

They remain our friends, and Richard's art—the wooden coin box that Jay painted under his tutelage—is still the daily depository for my coins, a constant reminder of the presence of two truly dear people in our and Jay's life.

16
Authentic Social Security

It is appropriate at this point to tell about Jay's life in the community before and after Anne and Richard become part of his and our lives. The story about his life in the community is about what Ann and I call "authentic social security."

Jay has a job; he lives in his own home; and he has stability in his housemates. He is receiving modest financial support from the Social Security system. There is security in his life, security that has come from hard work and deep commitment by many people.

We do not know, however, just how much security Jay has. Over time, we learn just how much and conclude that Jay's greatest social security derives from his simply living in his community and becoming known to ordinary people who are willing to be extraordinary for his sake.

Lost and Found

Tom Allison, a graduate student, precedes Richard and Anne as Jay's housemate. He believes Jay can learn how to take the bus from his home to work, and he begins to train Jay, first accompanying him and gradually fading his presence.

Within a month or so, Jay is independent in taking the bus. He boards the bus a half-block from his home, gets off at a campus stop, crosses a street, walks through one building (down one stair), crosses a lawn, enters another building, takes the elevator up to a bridge connecting that building to yet another, and then walks through that building until he reaches the wing where he works, and takes an elevator down one floor to his office.

We meet with the bus dispatcher, tell him who Jay is, bring along photographs of Jay that also set out his home telephone number, our home and office telephone numbers, his address, and Tom's cell phone number.

He sits behind co-eds and we worry whether he will pull their pony-tails, but he doesn't. We worry about whether he will board the wrong bus on his route home, but he doesn't—except once.

One day Jay boards the wrong bus when returning from work. He fails to arrive home at the usual time. Tom calls us, and we call the dispatcher, in a panic. "We are Jay Turnbull's parents. Jay got on a bus but did not arrive home. He's lost. What can you do? What can we do?"

The dispatcher remembers us and Jay.

"Don't worry. I'll call the bus drivers and find who has him. I'll call right back."

Moments later, the dispatcher calls us. "I've got him; he's on the wrong bus. I've told the driver to stop the bus and wait for me. I'll get Jay and take him home. And let me tell you, Jay was not lost. We wouldn't let Jay get lost. He was just misplaced."

We have given Jay to the community, and the community has been his safety net.

The Watcher

Later that same year, Jay leaves his house to go to his bus stop, adjacent to an elementary school. He walks slowly, somewhat depressed, and misses his bus. He stands and waits. A car pulls up. The driver speaks to Jay. Jay gets into the car, which drives away.

Across the street, Christie Jewell, a teacher, stands at her window, having coffee before classes begin. She looks out every morning and sees Jay. He does not know her, but she and her husband know Jay and us.

Christie calls us in a panic. "Jay got into a brown car, not the bus. I've called the police and given them a description of the car. No, I don't have a license plate number and didn't really get a good look at the driver."

We call Jay's housemate. There is no answer. Tom owns a car, but we don't recall its color.

Within a few minutes, Jay arrives at work. We ask, "Where have you been?"

He answers, "In car. With Tom."

We call Christie and tell her that Jay is alright. We thank her profusely. She is modest, "I watch Jay every morning to make sure he gets onto the bus. I hope you don't mind. Jim [her husband] says such nice things about him, and so I keep an eye on him. Is that OK?"

Is it OK? Of course it is.

We have put Jay out into our community and created a predictable and frequent presence for him there. We are not surprised his fellow citizens have safeguarded him.

Red Cards and Green Cards

It is 1992 and Jay has been living in his home on Hilltop Drive for three years. He needs someone to drive him to work daily, and his roommates are not always available. Ann meets with the owner of the local taxi-cab company, Shirley Bennett.

Ann describes Jay and what he needs—simply a regular pick-up and return. Then she describes what *she* needs—reassurances that the driver will not rob Jay or burglarize his home, not treat him disrespectfully, assault him, even sexually abuse him, or kidnap him. Shirley listens intently, nodding with understanding as Ann enumerates her fears. Ann finishes, in tears.

Shirley reaches into her desk drawer and pulls out three or four pieces of red construction paper and three or four of green construction paper. She hands the green ones to Ann and keeps the red ones. Ann is puzzled, for Shirley has not said a word. Ann asks, "Shirley, I don't understand. What are you doing?"

Shirley responds,

"Oh, Ann, don't you see? I wake up every morning hoping I can do something good for someone. I take their red cards of worry and give back my green cards of helpfulness. Here is my green card of understanding, my green card of friendship, and my green card of helpfulness."

Ann is stunned, silent. Shirley continues, "Come back tomorrow. I'll have a solution for Jay and you by then."

Ann returns the next day. Sitting in Shirley's office is a driver, a down-at-heels man who has tried to retain his respectability; life has been hard for him, that much is obvious.

"Ann and Bill, I want you to meet each other. Ann, I told Bill what Jay needs and about Jay and about your concerns. I have never before designated a driver for any passenger, but I am doing so today. Is that alright with you, Ann? With you, Bill?"

Ann assents. Bill pauses and asks a question, "Shirley, why did you choose me?"

Shirley answers, "Because, Bill, you need a friend as much as Jay does."

For nearly three more years, Bill and a line of trustworthy successors become Jay's drivers. The red and green cards have been exchanged, symbols of caring and being cared-for.

Kindness of Near-Strangers

It is spring, 1997. Richard and Anne are living with Jay, who is in one of his deeply depressed states. Despite all of Anne's and Richard's coaxing, he will not rise from his bed. Anne must go to class, and Richard must do a quick and nearby errand, so he leaves their home for a few minutes—the shopping center is only two blocks away and Jay seems destined to remain in bed for the rest of the day.

While Richard is absent, however, Jay rises, walks out of his home in his pajamas, walks up the street to one of the most heavily trafficked streets in town, and follows its sidewalk toward the university, about a half-mile to a mile away. Confused and depressed, he leaves the sidewalk and now is in traffic lanes. Cars swerve around him.

One passes him, pulls onto the sidewalk, and stops. Its driver remains in the car, the passenger exits, goes to Jay and coaxes him out of the middle of the road and into her car. She asks him where he is going. He says "Haworth Hall," the building where he works at the university. She, a student, knows where that building is. She coaxes him into her car, drives him there and accompanies him as he takes the elevator to up one floor and walks to his desk. He is still wearing his pajamas.

We ask her, "Who are you? What happened?"

She tells us what happened and then answers, "I see Jay every Saturday when he comes to visit his grandfather at his grandfather's apartment. I am the receptionist. Jay always greets me. I just had to help him."

By connecting Jay and Ann's father for weekly visits, we

inadvertently created a safety net for Jay. Bringing him into his community creates community around him.

The Postman's Daughter

It is spring during one of the years when Jay was living with Pat and Corey. Jay is in the living room, looking out onto Hilltop Drive. He sees a young girl, approximately three or four years old, walking down the sidewalk. She is with her father. Inexplicably, he bolts out of the house, runs toward the girl and begins to pull her hair. She yells, and Richard and Anne run to her rescue.

Richard and Anne have taken Jay inside, where Anne is trying to calm him, for he has just begun the down-turn from this episode. Richard goes outside and explains and apologizes to the man, a postman. The postman tolerates a short explanation and then takes his daughter home.

Richard calls me and I come to Hilltop Drive and instantly go to the postman's home. I fear the worst—that the man will have called the police and Jay will become involved in the criminal justice system.

I explain about Jay and his disabilities and moods, and I begin to apologize and offer to cover all expenses, if any, for any medical or psychological care his daughter needs.

The postman hears me out and then says, "Don't worry about it, Mr. Turnbull. I've delivered mail to Jay many times and know he's an OK person, and my daughter's frightened, that's all. She'll get over it."

I learn two lessons: never let Jay be alone, and contact my lawyer for advice on whether to contact the local police to alert them to the fact that Jay has a disability. Richard and Anne promise: they will keep Jay within sight whenever he is awake. The lawyer advises to lay low, for, if Jay becomes involved in the justice system, we will do a "diversion agreement." Meanwhile, we are to keep a careful record of all we do to manage Jay's behaviors and to protect others from him.

I wonder, What enabled the postman to forgive? Was it that he had seen the "other" Jay? That we had not isolated Jay, not kept him in congregate care, where he would have been guarded and segregated? Years later, we meet the postman's daughter, now a teenager. She has not forgotten, but she has forgiven.

Vouching

Jay works on the third floor at Haworth Hall. One floor below the one where he works, there is a speech-language clinic; and two floors below, there are classrooms for infants and toddlers with and without disabilities.

One day, Jay enters a pre-school classroom. He stands and looks at the youngsters. The undergraduates who work with the children become frightened; a stranger, and a strange-looking one at that, is in their midst. Their graduate student supervisor calls the campus police, who arrive within minutes. Jay remains standing; he has touched no one, approached no child.

Two policemen surround him and walk him out of the classroom. By now, Jay is the center of commotion. Someone who knows he is our son calls us, and we run down two flights of stairs to be with Jay, worried whether he has hurt anyone and whether he would be arrested and taken into custody.

One of the policemen has his arm over Jay's shoulder and is talking to him; both are grinning. We approach. The policeman introduces himself.

"I am Officer Sylvester Birdsong, and I was the security guard at the high school when Jay was there. I've told everyone what a great guy he is and not to worry. We're not going to do anything except write up a report. Jay's free to go home. He wouldn't harm a flea.

He's a good guy."

Jay had endeared himself to Officer Birdsong nearly a decade before, and now Officer Birdsong vouches for Jay. Jay does not enter the justice system; no judge hears a case against him, no prosecutor and defense lawyer negotiate a diversion agreement. It is enough that Jay has a friend.

Safety in the "Cheers" Connection

We have learned what it takes to increase Jay's joy quotient. It is to respond to his need for levity and laughter. Neither is possible without people, and thus comes a lesson about joy and connections.

During the 1990s and early into the first decade of the twenty-first century, one of Jay's favorite television shows is "Cheers." It portrays habituees of a bar in Boston, aptly named "Cheers."

Jay develops his "Cheers" connections. They are at his favorite restaurants. They are among his colleagues at work. They are with his and our friends at Plymouth Church. He gives his special handshake to his friends, and when he raises a toast at dinner parties, he says, "Cheers," mimicking me.

Places, people, gestures, and phrases create connections. Life becomes cheerful; a fictional bar in Boston becomes a reality in a dozen places in Lawrence. Among those places is The Free State Brewery, in downtown Lawrence.

Richard Gaeta and Anne Guthrie weekly take Jay to that bar-restaurant. There, Jay becomes a regular; this boisterous micro-brewery becomes a "Cheers" site—a place where everyone knows your name, at least those who count. Among those who meet and befriend Jay is the brewery's manager, Alex Hamilton.

On a regular "Free State" night, Richard is out of town. Yielding to Jay's insistence on routine, Anne takes him there for dinner. Alex charges Jay for a single soft-drink but gratuitously fills his glass as Jay gulps one and then another and yet another.

Now Jay must use the bathroom. He knows where it is, makes his way through the crowd, and returns. Within a minute, Alex appears and asks Anne, "Is Jay OK?"

Puzzled, Anne answers, "Yes, of course, but why do you ask?"

Alex explains,

"I went into the men's room just after Jay did, and when I got there, I saw one of the patrons pushing Jay up against the wall and ready the throttle him. I shouted, 'Leave him alone. That's JT!' The man released his grip on Jay's throat and explained, 'He was looking at me in a funny way.' I responded, 'Jay has autism, he's not a homosexual, and don't you ever touch him again. And tell your friends, too: Jay is my friend.'"

The man left the restaurant immediately, abashed and ashamed.

We ask Alex, "How did you know about Jay? What is it about you that made you his protector?"

He answers, "Oh, when I was in elementary school, we had gym and music classes with students like him. He had already moved on in school, but I learned that kids like him aren't all that different. They just need more help than the rest of us."

The "Cheers" connection—giving Jay away to the community, ensuring he is a regular in a few key places—safeguards Jay. And integration in school makes it possible to "give away" and expect that kind of "more help" that Alex provided.

Jay's greatest social security is his circle of friends.

17
Jay at Plymouth Church

Jay was baptized in the Roman Catholic Church, for that was the church of my ex-wife and her family. But he has never attended, for my ex-wife and I, being of different sects, chose not to attend any church.

With Ann, however, there is a different norm. I am a high-church Episcopalian and Ann is a Methodist. In Chapel Hill, we belonged to the Chapel of the Cross, an Episcopal church. When we come to Lawrence, we join Plymouth Congregational Church.

It was the first church established in the Kansas territory, in the mid-1850s, built by New England pioneers determined to bring their religion, education, and abolitionist fervor to the territory. Its present sanctuary and balcony were built by 150 members to accommodate nearly ten times that number; its design is in the manner of the New England Congregational churches, simple, unadorned, and straightforward.

The Power

We attend church regularly, heading always for the next-to-last pew so Jay and I can leave the service unobtrusively for the restroom. To the left of us, in the same row of pews, is Sue Hill, my senior by about a decade. We are acquaintances, nothing more.

A few weeks after Jay's funeral, Ann and I return to Plymouth, sit in our usual pew, and are lost in our thoughts about Jay. It is time to exchange the Peace Greeting; we reach over to give it to Mrs. Sue Hill. She tells us, "I never spoke the Lord's Prayer out loud when Jay was here. I always wanted to hear him say it. He said it so intently."

And so he did, coming to the phrase "For thine is the Power," and pronouncing the "P" with power, pushing the sound out of his mouth. Everyone near us can hear Jay. Even Peter Luckey, our pastor, some twenty pews away, picks up on it and smiles his way through the rest of the Prayer.

High Holy-days

As much as Jay becomes agitated by holidays—he wishes them to be over so he may return to his routine—he also knows how to celebrate them, especially Christmas. Christmas Eve at Plymouth Church has its absolutely rigid routine: hymns, lessons, sermon, and then, at the end, the congregation's soft singing of "Silent Night," the congregates holding lighted candles.

Jay sings it, but is not silent. We try to mute him, and succeed only when, in the second and third choruses, it is time to light the candles and hold them aloft. Then, Jay is silent, but instead of holding his candle high, he blows out the flame, his and ours, too. The symbolism by-passes him; his concern is for safety.

At Easter, Jay is uncontainable. He conducts the choir and brass band, both arms pumping to the rhythm, his voice loud on the "Alleluia" choruses.

He could not read the word "God" even if it were printed in large letters alone on a page. But he knows God; he has the Spirit. He receives and emits it. Jay is simplicity itself: free of knowledge, he yet knows in a different way.

The Plymouth Covenant

Our church services always close with the entire congregation reciting the church's covenant. In it we commit to pursue justice, labor for knowledge, seek the reign of peace, and celebrate our shared humanity.

Jay insists on his version of justice, of what is due to him; and we advocate for it. He pushes us to pursue the truth of our lives, and we find that truth: in service to a cause. He insists on knowledge, and we develop and transmit it. He seeks peace—his own kind, the harmony of his behaviors and his inner nature; in time, he and we find that peace. And, most of all, he celebrates shared humanity, creating community and bringing disparate people together.

The Long Goodnight Prayer

Jay has a remarkably strong long-term memory. The proof lies in the prayers he recites. Some nights, it is as though his memory is blocked; he prays for people now in his life, a "short list" or "A-list" as it were. Other nights, it is as though all of his memory circuits are open; he is "firing" and "hot."

On those nights, he recites the "Lord's Prayer" and then begins the lineage litany—the recitation of the names of his friends from long ago, a line-up of to-be-blessed beloveds.

First, Jay's family, including Granddaddy Turnbull, "in Heaven with Baby Jesus, smoking a pipe;" then Grandmommy Ruthie, singing "Bye Bye Blackbird;" then Ann's father, A-Dad, singing "You get a line, I get a pole, we go down to the crawdad hole."

Then Amy and Kate, next Rahul, Amy's husband, and our grandchildren, Dylan, Cameron, and Maya, and then Kate's boyfriend Chip. Thereafter, Jay reaches far back in time. He remembers his house-parents and roommates from his group home in Massachusetts. Then he blesses his Chapel Hill teachers and friends.

At this point, he has named more than two dozen people.

The "short" version of the prayers can last a minute or two; the long one, a good quarter of an hour.

We have no idea what unlocks his memory, but we know that relationships count in his life and we join Jay in prayer, giving thanks to the many people who have blessed him and us.

Jay's prayer litany—whether the short or long version—has a uniform concluding request. When he has exhausted the list of named individuals whom he asks God to bless, Jay always says, "And God bless all the good people."

Ann's father, A-Dad, observes, "Jay won't pray for any S.O.B."

Indeed that is so, but Jay knows there are many good people. He cannot remember all of them, and he cannot anticipate which of them will come into his life. But he knows enough to bless them all.

He is a collector of those from his past, present, and future.

Uniformed for God

Jay has a uniform for all high occasions, holidays, photographs, church, birthdays, and transition parties: white shirt, red tie, blue blazer, gray or khaki pants, and dark shoes. He wears these at his transition party from our home to the adult agency, at Amy's wedding, and at Amy's and Kate's graduation parties. He wears them to church (and his funeral); no other clothing is fit for worship—he refuses all alterations to this, his "dress" uniform.

The Salvation Army Christmas Bucket

It is Christmas season, 2008. Shelby Tasset, Jay's job coach and friend, takes Jay to Hy-Vee, a large grocery store, to shop. She drops him off at the front door and parks the car. She sees him approach and then walk away from the Salvation Army bell ringer. She asks the bell ringer if everything is OK. With tears in his eyes he answers,

"He opened up his wallet and gave me everything in it."

Jay is following Tom Riffel's example, for Tom always opens his wallet and gives the bell ringer money every day when they shop at the local supermarket. Jay usually carries $8 in his wallet—part of his daily wage, paid in cash as the immediate reinforcer for working well. He gives it all away. He does not understand much about money but he totally understands about giving to others.

Beyond Church: Gentleman Jay, A Gift to Our Communities

Jay's great skills are his gentlemanliness, his obviousness about what he likes and whom he cares for and does not, his authenticity, his inability to feign and dissemble. He is an utterly honest person. He endears himself in part because of his social graces.

All the money spent on teaching him new skills would have been relatively useless for his inclusion in our communities if he had not also learned the social graces of being a gentleman—"gentleman Jay," as he called himself.

Ann and I have taught him his social graces: for life in Chapel Hill, it's knowing the "Tar Heel Fight Song;" for life everywhere, it's his cordial greeting of friends and strangers, and his table manners. Others teach him unique ways to connect with people. Corey Royer, the fraternity man who launched Jay into living in his own home, and Jay's sister Kate teach him a way to change his voice to emphasize the hard consonants and minimize the soft vowels—this "T-Talk" that so delights him and his inner circle of friends. Pat Hughes and Corey teach him the SAE handshake, which replaces the "high five" once he lives with them.

Instinctively, Jay knows that, when he uses the SAE handshake, he connects in a unique way with others. He usually declines to use an ordinary handshake, preferring the fraternity one. He then offers his own version of a "high five," rubbing the back of his right hand against the back of his partner's, repeating the gesture with his left hand, and finally ending the ritual with a snap of the fingers that Rahul taught him. We admonish, "Use your church handshake," referring to the regular way of shaking hands, emphasizing he should especially resort to this in church.

But Jay is adamant: my way or no shake at all. We are helpless to prevent him from using it. Some people "get it" from the beginning, following him easily; others struggle; but all remember him. He signals, "I am different but gentlemanly." He creates his own special connections to his community. He radiates beyond our church.

The stories that follow illustrate these special connections and, just as importantly if not more importantly, the power he had to transform people and the power others had to include and enjoy Jay. If ever proof were needed that we did right by him by giving him to our community, these stories provide the proof.

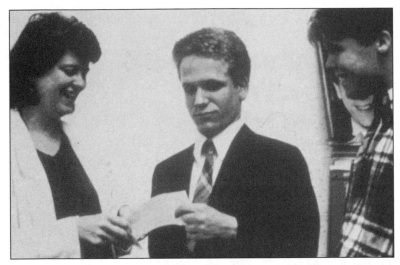

Jean Ann Summers, Jay, 21, and Pat Hughes, as Jay receives his first paycheck, University of Kansas, 1988

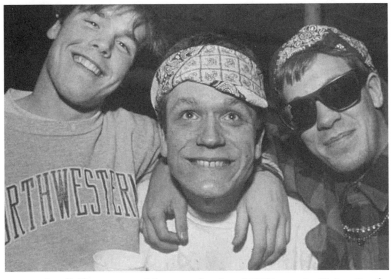

Pat Hughes (left), Jay, 22, and fraternity brother, SAE Fraternity, University of Kansas, 1989

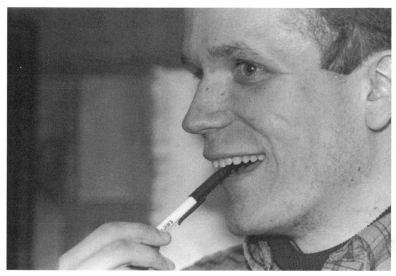

Jay, 22, Lawrence, Ks., 1989

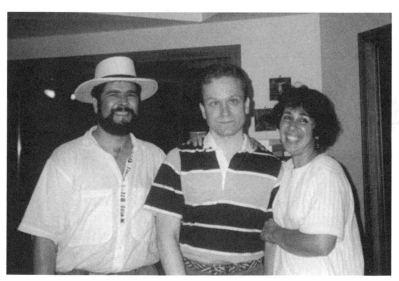

Jay, 23, with housemates Jesus and Shahla Rosales, Lawrence, Ks.,1990

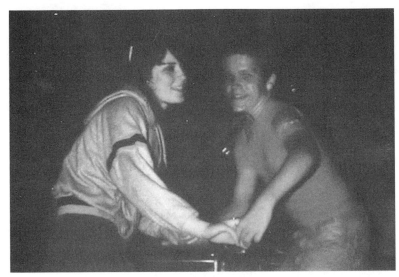

Jay, 15, with Suzanne Kiper Knowlton, summer camp, Carrollton, Ky., 1982

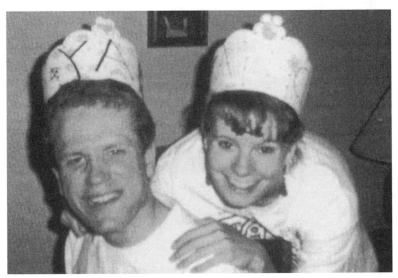

Jay, 23, at birthday party with Della Clayton, Lawrence, Ky., 1990

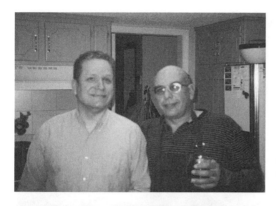

Jay, 25, with housemate Richard Gaeta, Lawrence, Ks., 1992

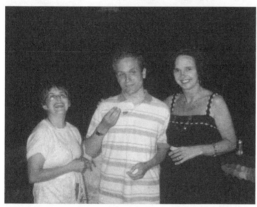

Jay, 26, with Dana Gates (left) and Ann (right), Lawrence, Ks., 1993

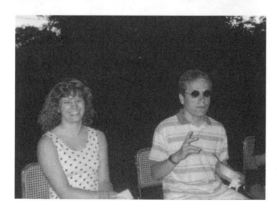

Jay, 26, at birthday party with Della Clayton, Lawrence, Ks., 1993

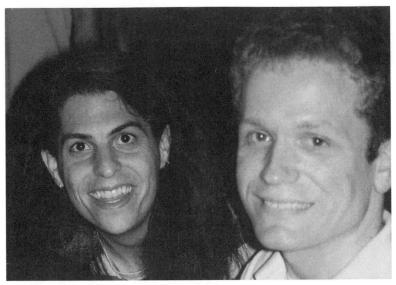

Jay, 29, with housemate Tom Allison, Lawrence, Ks., 1996

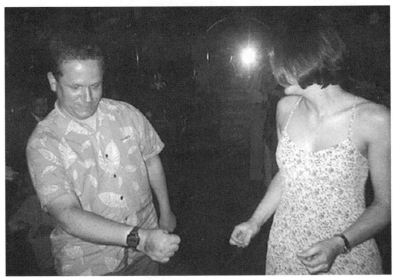

Jay, 29, with Sarah Eldredge, University of Kansas, 1996

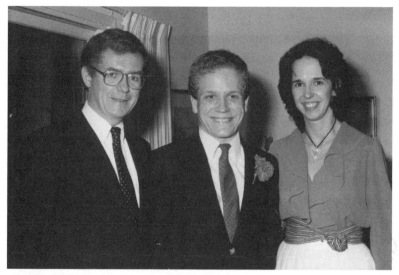

Rud, Jay, 30, and Ann, Lawrence, Ks., 1997

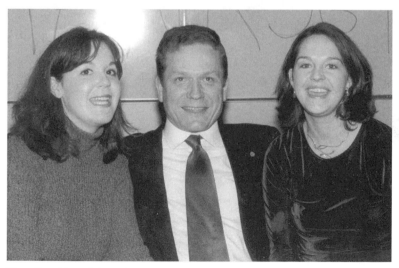

Kate, Jay, 30, and Amy, Lawrence, Ks., 1997

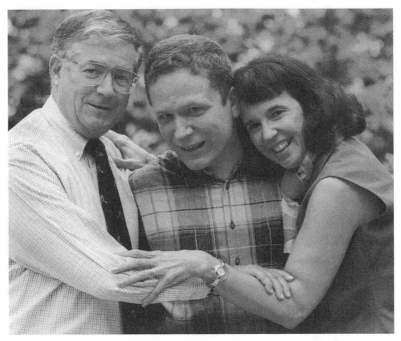

Rud, Jay, 32, Ann, Lawrence, Ks., 1999

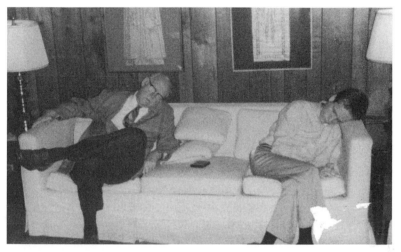

Jay, 22, with Ann's father, H. F. Patterson, or "A-Dad", doing their favorite activity, Lawrence, Ks., 1989

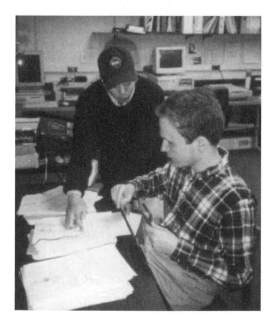

Jay, 32, with co-worker Richard Viloria, Beach Center on Disability, University of Kansas, 1999

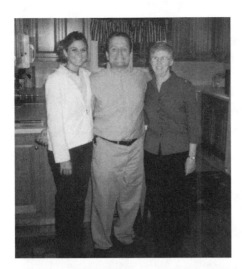

Jay, 32, with unidentified graduate student (left) and speech-therapy supervisor Jane Wegner (right), University of Kansas, 1999

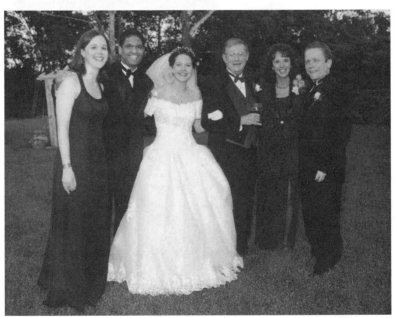

Kate, Rahul Khare, Amy, Rud, Ann, Jay , 33, at Amy and Rahul's wedding, Lawrence, Ks., 2000

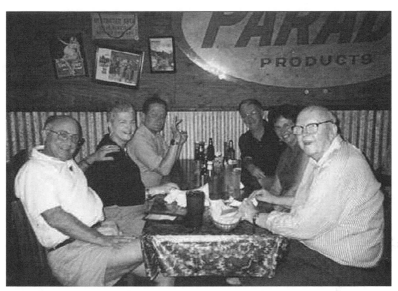

William Huguley (Ann's brother-in-law), Virginia ("Teo") Huguley (Ann's sister), Jay, 33, Rud, Ann, and Ann's father, H. F. ("A-Dad") Patterson, Lawrence, Ks., 2000

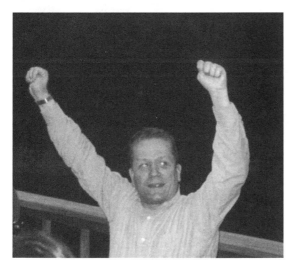

Jay, 33, celebrating, Lawrence, Ks., 2000

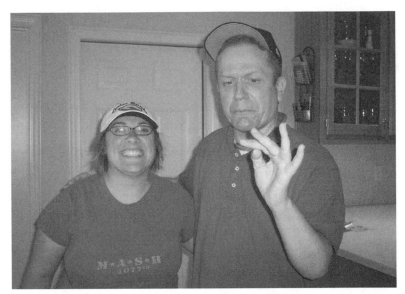

Jay, 36, with music therapist Gayla Berry, Lawrence, Ks., 2003

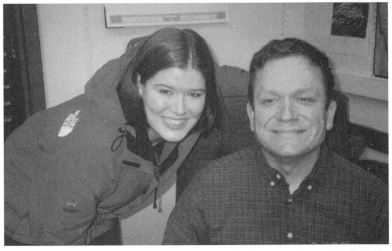

Jay, 37, with co-worker Lauren Priest, Beach Center on Disability, University of Kansas, 2004

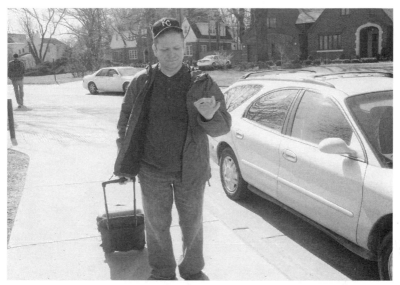

Jay, 37, delivering mail, University of Kansas, 2004

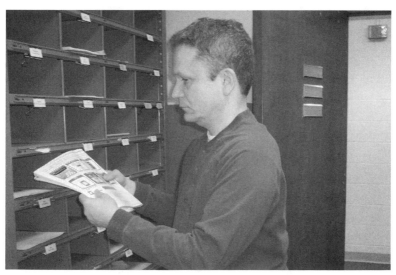

Jay, 37, sorting mail, Beach Center on Disability, University of Kansas, 2004

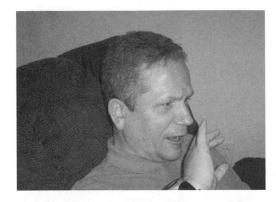

*Jay, 37, Lawrence, Ks.,
2004*

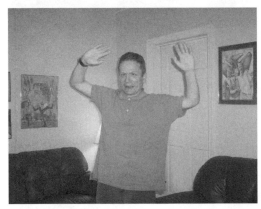

*Jay, 37, Lawrence, Ks.,
2004*

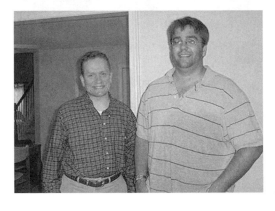

*Jay, 37, with co-worker
Tom Manthey, Beach
Center on Disability,
University of Kansas,
2004*

18

The Best Years of His Life
(2000–2009)

In a very real sense, Jay began his adult life with Mary Morningstar as his teacher in Bethesda, Maryland. He was twenty-one and finally learning how be in school—that is, in a given community—with students who did not have disabilities—metaphorically, to live an integrated life. His years with Pat and Corey, then Jesus, Shala, and Corey again, and then with a succession of housemates supported him to be even more part of the Lawrence community. We had concluded that he was at his most supported when living with Anne Guthrie and Richard Gaeta, and were more than a little distraught when they announced they were leaving after four years as Jay's housemates.

What to do now, who will replace them? It could not be Amy and Kate, both of whom were in school or college. Nor could Jay return to live with us—he would not want it, nor, in fact, would we. From being distraught we became anxious, more anxious, and exceedingly anxious.

We need not have worried. Laura Riffel relieved our concerns in ways we did not even imagine could occur.

Having earned her undergraduate and master's degree in education at Kansas State University, Laura enrolls to earn her doctorate at the University of Kansas, in the mid-1990s. To help support her while she is taking courses, Ann and I hire her to be Jay's job coach.

In the summer of 2001, Laura approaches us, knowing Richard Gaeta and Anne Guthrie are ready to leave after four years as Jay's housemates. "We want to live with Jay. We love him. We want him to have a good home."

The "we" includes her husband Tom, a retired civilian employee of the Army and, like Laura, a native Kansan.

We meet with them and readily agree. Having Tom and Laura means having their children. Indeed, when Tom and Laura leave for slightly over three years so she may work in Georgia, their son Bryan takes over as housemate. Two Riffels now become three and, in short order, five. Bryan involves his brother Brandon and sister Jessica as the support team for Jay.

When Bryan's muscular dystrophy makes it difficult for him to take care of Jay without additional support, and because Tom and Laura want to return to be with Bryan, Tom returns from Georgia, followed a few months later by Laura. Bryan remains constant in his friendship to Jay, always available to spend weekends with him. Nor does Brandon step back; indeed, he steps up, bringing his girlfriend Sarah Johnson (now his wife), his friend Bobby Young and Bobby's sister Andrea, and then distant cousins, especially Levi Braham and their friends, into Jay's life.

These young people take to Jay, and he to them; they develop their own games, their own codes and passwords to delight. A joyous crowd creates a joyous Jay. The joy quotient is as important as Jay's IQ and adaptive behaviors. The following stories make that simple point.

One caveat is in order. There are two kinds of humor about a family—inside and outside. Inside humor is what family members tell each other, delighting in the quirks and peculiarities of those whom they love. Outside humor is what family members tell non-family members. The former can be far less restrained than the latter. And it can seem, to outsiders, to diminish the dignity of the person who is the central focus of the inside humor.

What follows are inside-humor stories. They tell how Jay and people who were relative strangers to him—especially Tom, Bryan, and Brandon—became family to each other. They do not diminish Jay. Indeed, they dignify him by portraying his power to transform others and convert them to his life. Of course, they also dignify Laura, Tom, Bryan, and Brandon by telling how they, in idiosyncratic ways, entered Jay's life and were transformed by him. Tom says it best when he tells us, "Jay put the child back into me." They were among the many who put the dignity into Jay's life.

A Gourmet, the "Cheers" Connection, and Inclusion

In Lawrence, Jay becomes a bon vivant, a gourmet in Lawrence's rather modest restaurant scene. He goes to the Mad Greek on the same night every week and orders the same food, spaghetti, meatballs, and garlic bread. The proprietors, George and Peggy Kristos, tell their staff, "Give Jay a menu even though he does not read, and give him the dignity of ordering on his own even though you know he will order the same meal every time." They dignify him, refusing to infantilize him.

In other restaurants, there is similar acceptance. Proprietors, staff and regulars at other restaurants come to know Jay. They welcome him as Peggy has welcomed him—he's more than a customer, he's a friend.

Repetitive visits introduce Jay to other regulars. We regularize his routine, and we in turn regularize him. He becomes one of the regulars, an accustomed patron. Nothing about him stands out any more. He has found his "Cheers" places—those establishments where everyone knows your name and takes you in, just as you are. But being a regular in restaurants has its down-side.

Jay does not diet. Truth be told, he indulges himself. He splurges while in restaurants: pastas, heavy meats, and desserts are his regular diet. He snacks at home if Tom and Laura and we are not careful (as we all try to be) to not have snack-food at home: Tootsie Rolls, miniature peanut-butter cookies, Triscuits, frosted sugar cookies, Wheat Thins, and Oreo cookies. He has his favorite foods, none of which is diet-smart: meat loaf and gravy, Kentucky Fried Chicken, steaks on Sunday nights at our home, mashed potatoes with brown and white gravy (he is unwilling to chose one gravy over the other so we serve both), cheeseburgers, and ice cream.

The older he is, the larger he becomes. He loses weight when he is depressed; to restrict his eating when he is not depressed simply provokes a confrontation and possible eruptions. We yield, but we contain the quantity. He wins—his choice prevails. We win, too—to some degree, we determine the quantity.

Grace and Small Bites

It is customary for us to say Grace before dinner.

"Bless, oh Lord, these gifts to our use, and our lives to thy loving service. Give us grateful hearts and make us mindful of the needs of others, in Christ's name we pray. Amen."

Jay prefers a simpler Grace, the one we taught him, Amy, and Kate years before we began using the Grace I learned as a child. Being true to himself, Jay embellishes it. "God is great, God is good, let us thank Him for our food. Amen, amen, amen. Let's eat! Small bites!"

Whereupon he opens his mouth as wide as he can and takes in as much as he can. He has a concept of divinity and knows to be grateful but he has an appetite and does not adhere to his own admonitions.

The Censor

Long before Jay and the Riffel family join with each other, Jay started speech-language therapy. One aspect of the therapy was teaching Jay how to communicate with others—to be a partner in a conversation. And part of that teaching was making sure he would not use vulgarity.

Jay and I watch TV together on Sunday nights. We favor "The Sopranos," a "gangster" drama in which the characters use the "F" word in nearly every sentence. Jay always interrupts, "Don't say that word."

I lose half of the dialogue, for Jay is ever the gentleman. But it is no matter—being with him is enjoyment enough.

When Laura becomes lost while driving with him, she often curses, "Damn." He interjects, "Don't say that word."

And then, mimicking her, "We're turning around" (to find the correct way to their destination).

He is the forgiving but correcting gentleman.

And because he is a gentleman, Jay almost never swears. One day, however, Sarah Johnson hears Jay say "damn," a nearly-first time use of vulgarity. She asks, "Jay, what words don't we say?"

Jay answers, giving five or so of the "no-no" words, having learned from the speech-therapy students and us, while watching television with him, that he should not say them. Shocked, Sarah never asks that question again.

The Naked Night-Walker

Brandon, Tom and Laura's son, returns to Lawrence after year of working in Colorado, ready to start his studies at the university. He has not met Jay before now.

It is early on the first morning he spends at Jay's home, sleeping upstairs in a guest bedroom. It is sometime past midnight but not yet at the hour when night recedes to the dawn.

Brandon is restless and hungry. He leaves his bedroom, goes to the kitchen, and peers into the refrigerator.

He hears footsteps and turns around. Jay is carrying his sheets and pajamas, which he has soiled, to the laundry room, traversing the kitchen. He is totally naked and obviously pleased with himself, grinning broadly—he's taking care to clean up after himself. "Dad! Dad!" screams Brandon.

Tom rises from his sleep and comes downstairs. Father and son stand in the kitchen. Brandon is nearly shocked and clearly at a loss for words. Tom, is nonplussed. Jay is utterly oblivious that anything is amiss. Unashamed of his nakedness, Jay leaves the laundry room, walks through the kitchen, and returns to his bedroom. He now is fully exposed because he is not carrying his sheets or bedclothes.

Brandon tells Tom, "That was not the best way to meet Jay for the first time!"

Tom, Laura, and Brandon warn other overnight guests.

"Jay may wet his bed. We usually don't have overnight guests. He will undress and take his clothes to the laundry room. If you have any problems with this, if it makes you uncomfortable, it is best to stay upstairs or turn away."

Staying upstairs or turning away does not always work. Sarah Johnson, Brandon's girlfriend and soon-to-be-wife, spends the night at Jay's house; Tom and Laura are away. She awakes before Jay and is in the kitchen. Jay has wet his bed. He removes his clothes, puts them onto his wet sheets, strips his bed, and walks into the kitchen, carrying his sheets and clothes to the washing machine. Sarah exclaims, "Oh my God, Jay, I don't want to picture you like that!"

Jay laughs hysterically. Her alarm is his glee. He is not ashamed of his nakedness. Indeed, he is acutely unaware of sex differences.

Most of his care-givers are men, but a few are women. They regard him as a nurse would regard a male patient—the bathing is a professional act of cleanliness and a personal act of kindness. Jay is unconscious of gender differences; he knows men and women are different, but he does not know the genital differences. Unwitting of that distinction and its social connotations, he does not know not to expose himself to just anyone. But he does know that he must clean up after himself. There are trade-offs. Within the family, some are easier to make than others.

Obsessions, Games, and Adjustments

Jay's OCD means that everything has its place and must be in that place. Tom converts Jay's obsessions into games.

The dish towel must hang on the handle of the oven, flush right. When Tom moves it to the center of the handle, Jay returns to the kitchen to move it to the far right. Tom moves it again. Jay glares at Tom, who repositions the towel, this time where Jay wants it. Jay says, "Fine," grins, and leaves the kitchen.

Tom turns his attention to the dog's food/water and bell, or to light switches. He moves them to their irregular positions; Jay returns them to their regular ones. Jay allows no deviations.

But now, it is not a matter of obsession and compliance. Instead, two grown men are playing a game and delighting each other as they do. They find a way of connecting, of making each interact jokingly with the other. Levity enters their lives. We yield to him on the small things in life, as we do our alchemy of making light of what is otherwise heavy for Jay. Tom has found the way. The rest of us mimic him.

Laura, too, learns how to deal with Jay's perseverance. When he goes on and on and on about a dinner of meatloaf and gravy, she holds up a finger and silences him, "OK, one time, we are having meatloaf."

He holds up one finger and no longer repeats "meatloaf." He gets what he wants—a promise for a meal, and Laura gets what she wants—a question posed and answered just once.

Reinforcers

Tom and Laura find sure-fire reinforcers that entice Jay away from and often out of OCD and mild depressions.

Jay likes to sleep late. Often, too late: there are errands to do and a job to carry out. Laura finds a way to make Jay rise from bed even when he does not want to.

When he stays in bed too long, Laura, in high heels, descends the uncarpeted stairs from her study to his room. The stairs are immediately outside his bedroom door. He cannot fail to hear her coming. Click, click, click go her heels; Jay knows she is coming for him. Not wanting to displease her, he rises. In her words, "I'm now the warden, the drill sergeant, not Jay's own Mary Poppins, his ever-cheerful elder."

Tom, too, finds ways to prompt Jay out of bed. He gives him choices about what to eat: eggs, waffles, pancakes, Raisin Bran, oatmeal. When the first choice approach does not work, Tom offers another. If it too fails, and a few thereafter, Tom asks, "Do you want liver and onions for breakfast?"

Jay has never had that meal, but he senses he would not like it and moves quickly out of bed. Choice-making empowers Jay, but trickery has its role, too.

Tom uses other approaches. He enters Jay's bedroom and says, "Good morning, Jay, time to get up." Jay responds, "Five more minutes." Or, "Pretty soon." Or, "I'm fine." Or, "Later." Tom responds, "We can't say 'Pretty soon'—I don't want to hear that.

How about five more minutes." He returns in two; Jay usually pops out of bed.

Jay can recite the holidays of the year, in order, but he cannot tell time. All he knows is that he has bought some time. That is enough for him—the small victory counts, the amount of time does not. Jay wins. So does Tom. No big trade-off is necessary.

When Jay persists in staying in bed, refusing all other blandishments or offers of an unpalatable breakfast, Tom says, matter-of-factly, "OK, no hotel next week." Jay leaps out of bed, repeats loudly "Brown hotel, brown hotel," and heads straight for the bathroom. Bryan and other young people escort him to the hotel. They too want a break in their routine, a mini-vacation. It's win-win time again.

When Jay has just had his weekend at the motel and is still recalcitrant about rising to work, Tom asks, "What Would Uncle Ruddy Say?" An "Uncle Ruddy" (my childhood name was Ruddy) from them was a sufficient prompt for him.

Tom often tells Jay, when he will not get out of bed, "OK, Mister, feet on the floor." It is one of my old phrases; it seems to work. I regularly use it when he is at work but locked into a temporary and mild depression. Tom adopts it for his own use. Jay's engagement beats withdrawal, and any phrase that gets Jay going is a good one.

Just as there is a morning routine, so too is there one for evenings. Laura often puts Jay to bed, saying, "Night Night, Sleep Tight, Don't let the bed bugs…"

Jay interrupts, giggling, "Bite, bite, bite."

If he goes to bed before Laura has a chance to say it, she stands outside his door and knocks. She asks whether she may enter. Sometimes Jay says yes and sometimes no. If he admits her, she opens the door and says the "night night." But if he denies her admission, she remains outside and says the refrain through the door and hears him giggle. All is well that ends well.

He knows he belongs to the Riffel family. Tom and Laura's daughter Jessica marries in the summer of 2007. Jay is a groomsman. He spends the afternoon dancing, kissing the girls, and eating. Jessica makes sure he is the first in the buffet line, after her and her husband Scot. Jay was already headed to the buffet, his instinct for food overriding the good manners of waiting for the bride and groom and their family. But he understands he is family, and Jessica and Scot treat him exactly so.

Within the Riffel family, the delight in Jay—just being with him, regardless of how he behaved—trumps any distress associated with his challenging or idiosyncratic behaviors.

Gas

It is a physiological fact: the human body creates gas that must be expelled. Among the Riffels, Jay's gas becomes a matter of amusement. One story makes the point.

Sarah Johnson takes Jay shopping. Rather than roam the aisles, Jay sits on a chair next to an older man. The older man looks askance at Jay, noticing he has walked differently and talks to himself—Jay's habit when he is feeling "up" and satisfied with himself. Jay in turn looks at his elder, rolls twice toward his right, and gasses the old man twice. The man, having endured these blasts, leaves and Jay sits alone, master of his domain.

Sarah tells us, "Jay always rolled to the right and once he started rolling, there was no stopping him." Sarah implores him in vain, "When you are with other people, do not pass gas."

Jay rolls nonetheless.

Sarah—like Tom, Laura, and Brandon—admits she is helpless to prevent this biological imperative. The who, what, when, where, and how of gassing becomes a topic of humor. Jay himself gets a kick out of it—he knows he is about to do wrong, he does wrong, he smiles, and then he apologizes. Good manners add some salvation to a social offense.

"Whoo Whoo Whoo"

Jay often expresses his delight by a phrase he learned from his sisters when they cheered or applauded an entertainer.

Brandon and his friend Bobby Young bring Jay to their apartment every Saturday afternoon, prepare his lunch, and let Jay do what he most wants to do—take a nap. Brandon or Bobby brings Jay his favorite blanket, lays it over his head, and begins to tuck Jay in. Jay flips the blanket up and tells them, "My feet," whereupon Brandon or Bobby tucks his feet under the blanket, but not first without tickling them. Jay, Brandon, and Bobby conclude the routine in harmony: "Whoo, whoo, whoo."

Sarah, Brandon, and Jay spend a weekend in the Honeymoon Suite at a Lawrence motel. The trip is one of Jay's "reward visits" to "the brown hotel." They sign in, causing no little consternation to the receptionist, whose quizzical face declares she is wondering who will do what to whom. They enter the suite and see a red, heart-shaped bathtub. Jay laughs and declares, "Whoo, whoo, whoo." There is one king-sized bed; Jay sees it and giggles. He sleeps on the cot that night.

Not every one of Jay's answers is appropriate for the circumstance. Sarah comes for music therapy on the night the KU men are competing in the televised national basketball championship game. Everyone is excited. Sarah asks, "JT, what is everyone going to be watching tonight?" Anticipating regularity, Jay answers, "Andy Griffith."

Picking Your Battle

Jay's IQ is such that he often nearly succeeds in figuring out how to con people. "Nearly" is the key word.

Speaking about the cookies Jay wants to eat, but should not, after returning from work and before dinner, Tom observes, "If you want to hide something, hide it in a low drawer because he doesn't want to bend down."

In the same vein, Brandon induces Jay to exercise before going to bed. "You can have your M&M's when you come up and give me twenty sit-ups."

Jay lies down, does one sit-up, and counts off the next five, "10, 11, 12, 18, 19. Finished. M&M time!"

Tom uses the same inducement, but Jay changes the numbers, "9, 10, 11, 14. Finished." and gets the same result—it's M&M time.

Tom and Jay often watch television at night, usually in the living room on the second floor of Jay's home, where Tom and Laura have their living quarters, separate from Jay's, downstairs. Tom keeps popcorn and peanuts upstairs, snacks for their TV time together.

Tom asks Jay, "Do you want popcorn?" Tom fetches some for Jay. The next night, same routine. The third night, Tom does not pose the question. Jay waits for it. And waits. And finally says, "That popcorn sure was good, that popcorn was good, that popcorn was good…"

Tom hears him out a few more times and offers the popcorn.

Tom reflects on the story, "With JT, you pick your battles. You don't pick very many of them, but you pick a few."

Popcorn was not one of them. Getting out of bed was.

Others' Joy Quotients

Jay's ability to integrate into his community derives from his modeling of others; we all set examples for him, and he learns to duplicate our behavior. That is not always good, nor are we always the best examples for him. Good or not, just as the Riffels and we contribute to Jay's joy quotient, he contributes to theirs and ours. A few stories make the point.

Hand Gestures

Brandon tries to un-teach Jay a hand gesture he has learned from watching the movie, *Indiana Jones*. He sees its star, an American, raise his fist, his middle finger extended, when hearing "Heil, Hitler." Jay associates bad people with the middle finger. Now, he wants to use it whenever a TV character is obviously bad, often adding "Heil, Hitler" as he flips off the evil character.

Tom and Jay encounter one of the stars of the university's national basketball championship team of 2008. Jay is stereotyping with his right hand, holding his fore-finger and thumb together while vigorously flapping his other three fingers. The young player, an African American, stares at Jay. Tom asks if there is a problem. The young man answers, "I'm trying to figure out if he's doing gang symbols."

Tom and Sarah, Brandon's now-wife, explain it is hard to drive when Jay wants to do his special handshake when being transported. They become one-handed drivers. Jay will not quit until he gets the shake, once and again.

Brandon asks Jay when his hands are flying, "What does Bryan say to do with your hands?" Jay answers, "Fold 'em," and he does.

The Helper

Sarah is looking frantically for her eyeglasses. She asks Jay where he has seen them. Jay puts her at ease, "Your glasses are on your hair."

Brandon's routine includes taking the dog, TJ, for walks. He cannot find the dog's leash and begins to obsess. Jay tells him, "Take the leash." Then he tells Brandon where it is, the master of everything in its place.

Complimenting

Gayla Berry, Jay's music therapist, takes JT to her parents' home for a party and dinner of chicken enchilada. He eats heartily, but not before giggling and complimenting them, "What a beautiful house you have."

He clears the table after he finishes eating, though they have not finished. No matter: They welcome him back often.

Socializing

Sarah takes Jay to a video store to rent a movie. JT is seated in a waiting area, two ladies are sitting on either side of him. He speaks to himself, "Mmm, that's right." The ladies talk across him, and Jay repeats, "Mmm, that's right."

Sarah approaches the ladies and, covering for Jay, asks, "Oh, JT, are you making friends?"

The ladies interrupt his answer: "He's such a sweet man."

Laura takes Jay to see Dr. Robert Batterson, Jay's psychiatrist, for a med-check. Dr. Batterson asks, "What's your favorite TV program?"

JT crosses his legs, leans back, and answers, "Well, perhaps...," modeling his psychiatrist perfectly.

Frugal and Complimentary

Brandon asks Jay, "Where do you want to go to eat, JT?" Jay, having learned well from Bryan, Brandon's older brother, answers, "Somewhere cheap."

Laura tells Jay, "I like your shirt."
He answers, "That's a compliment. I like yours, too."
He learns to give them.

His Way Only

Laura says, "If you flush the Post-it note down the toilet, you're not getting your eight dollars." (This is his daily "wage" at work—cash in hand).

Jay throws the note into the trash basket and demands his $8.00. He distinguishes between objects, not aims.

Tom addresses the fact that Jay's underpants often are visible, his shirt tucked into them. "Jay, you look like Dorkus McGorkus," Tom says.

Jay then pulls his shirt completely out of his pants, revealing his belly. Tom seeks a solution—buy low-rider underwear—but Jay pulls them up as high as possible. Tom gives up, "Dorkus has returned."

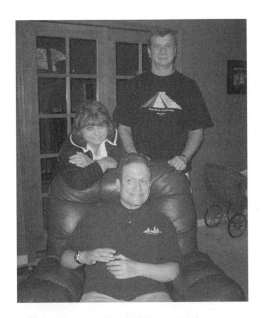

*Jay, 38, with housemates
Laura and Tom Riffel,
Lawrence, Ks., 2005*

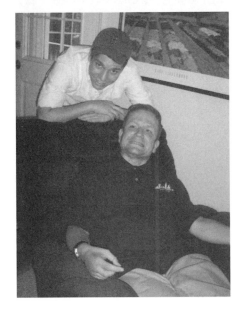

*Jay, 38, with Brandon Riffel,
2005*

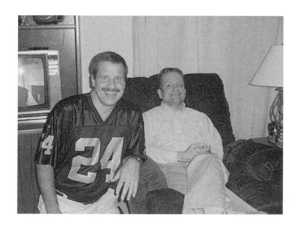

Jay, 39, with Bryan Riffel, 2006

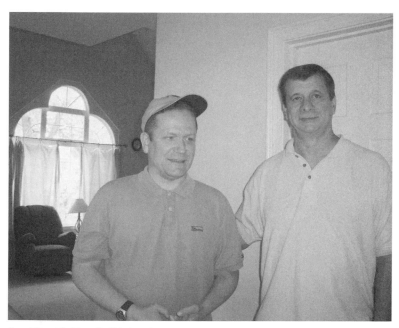

Jay, 39, with Tom Riffel, 2006

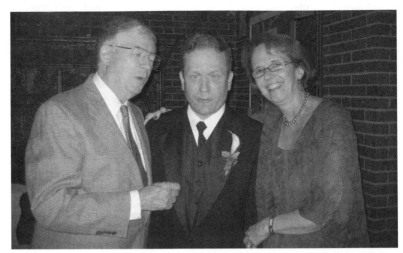

Rud, Jay, 40, and Ann, 2007

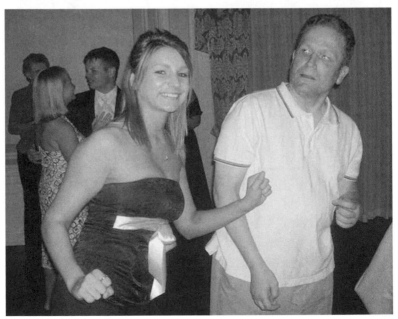

Jay, 40, with Sarah Johnson (Brandon Riffel's soon-to-be bride), 2007

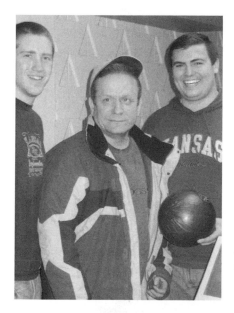

Jay, 40, with Andy and T. J.,
Kappa Sigma fraternity,
University of Kansas, 2007

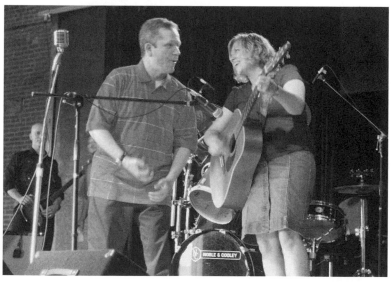

Jay, 40, with Sarah Nilleksela, at his birthday party, Lawrence, Ks., 2007

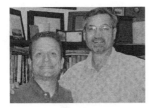

Jay, 40, with professor Mike Wehmeyer, Beach Center on Disability, University of Kansas, 2007

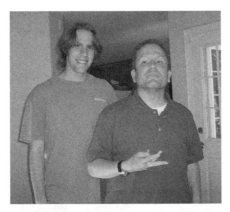

Jay, 40, with John Muller, Lawrence, Ks., 2007

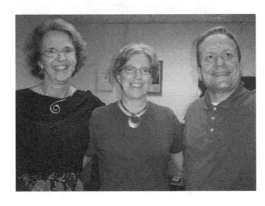

Ann, co-worker Lois Weldon, and Jay, 40, Beach Center on Disability, University of Kansas, 2007

19
The Last Touches

In the year and one-half before he dies, there are unexpected run-ups to Jay's death. They are the last touches, though we do not know it and could hardly have anticipated it.

Jay's 40th Birthday and Preludes to Funeral Music

The summer of 2007 comes, and in late June Jay celebrates his 40th birthday at a local bar, Abe and Jake's. We order food and consume it and beer. There is music; Jay and Sarah Niileksela lead us in song, and Judith Gross' husband, Tom Andrews, has brought a band that gives us dance music when it is not doing rock and roll and soul songs. Laura organizes a "Dollar Dance," charging all girls a dollar to dance with Jay, giving Jay the proceeds of his non-stop JT Shuffling. This is the last large collective celebration until the one on the day of his funeral. Joy precedes grief.

Implosion and Safety

The five months before Jay dies are unhappy for us professionally. Our core federal grant at the Beach Center expires in September, 2008. We compete for other grants, working outside of our field, and we fail in our efforts. Jay faces unemployment, the unraveling of his routine, the loss of his spending money. Jay is unaware, however, and is his "true" self, the magnetic, smiling, "fine" man. Our colleague Mike Wehmeyer comes to the rescue and hires Jay onto one of his grants. Mike also hires Jay's job coach, Shelby Tasset.

Some ten years earlier, we recruited Mike to be the associate director of the Beach Center. We shared an authorship with him on our textbook. He now reciprocates, without being asked. At Jay's funeral, Mike tells us all, "We are in the dignity business." He has given Jay safe harbor and simultaneously dignified him.

Granola Bars

Wendy Parent is affiliated with our Center. During Jay's daily mail run to her office, in another building, she offers him a granola bar; it is his snack, her token to assure his performance, and her gesture of love and respect. She presses us to secure job coaching, to develop a plan for Jay to save his earnings. She seeks to re-qualify Jay for vocational rehabilitation services and a newly authorized federal savings plan. The week before Jay dies, she tells us, "Jay has qualified." He was on a new path, but we did not know which one.

The First Filling, the Last Cleaning

At the suggestion of Jay's regular dentist, who has found a cavity (Jay's first), Tom and I take Jay to a pediatric dentist. It is summer, 2008. She sedates him for the filling, puts him into a small room made for young children to calm down in after they have been sedated. It is too small for him, and he senses trouble lies ahead. He perseverates about drinking a soft drink, which the dentist used to disguise the sedative.

She brings him to the treatment room. He is not fully under the effects of the drug. Nurses hover around, speaking loudly, as if he were deaf. He waves his arms; his eyes roll left to right and back again; he makes increasingly loud "whoop" noises.

Suddenly, he rises violently out of the dentist's chair and runs toward an exit door. He screams, pushes through the door, and runs across the lawn of the dentist's office. Tom and I follow him and manage to force him into Tom's car.

There, headed home, he begins to scream again, flap his hands, and hit his head. Tom is alone in the car; I am in my own car, alone, preceding him. I look into my rear-view mirror and see Tom reaching softly over to Jay to hold his hands and distract him by singing.

We arrive at Jay's home some ten minutes and four episodes later, and offer Jay a choice to sleep in his bed or on a living room couch. He chooses the couch, we cover him with a blanket, we move a glass-top table away from the couch, and we sit nearby, ready to restrain him if he begins to hurt himself. He falls into a deep sleep.

The dentist calls and reprimands me for taking Jay away while he is in her office. "He's my patient and I am responsible for him!"

"No," I answer, "I told you he could explode and how to medicate him before putting him into that baby's waiting room. It was too small for him. He knew something bad was going to happen. You didn't listen, and you have no right to tell me how to take care of my son."

A few months pass. I call Richard Viloria, one of Jay's former job coaches and now a pediatric dentist in Kansas City. He secures copies of Jay's X-rays and says he will arrange to treat Jay himself, but in an operating theatre and with another dentist. Jay will need full sedation, he thinks. The procedure with Richard is scheduled for several months in the future. I do not want to wait that long.

I call Jay's regular dentist, Charlie Kincaid, and hygienist, Jane

Getto. He reviews the X-rays and tells me to bring Jay to see him. I do. Tom is with me and Jay, as he has been every time Jay goes to the dentist.

Jay, Charlie, and Jane greet each other; they are old friends. Jay submits to what he believes is his usual cleaning. Tom and I are in the room with him. Sometimes Jay terminates the cleaning abruptly and early. Not this time. Charlie drills the cavity without using Novocain, fills it, and sends Jay on his way. The procedure takes about twenty minutes. Jay looks at Tom and me the entire time. We reassure him. He trusts Charlie and Jane, he trusts Tom and me.

This is his first filling. It also is his last. He goes to his death with a perfect set of teeth.

We Gather Together

Amy, Rahul, Dylan, Cameron, and Maya come to our home for Thanksgiving. Kate and Chip are here, too, the entire family in one place, in good spirits. Amy's children take over the house. Jay sits, amused by them, but still keeping his distance. He does not play with them, but when they come to him, he pats them softly on their heads. He is the essence of sweetness, calm amid the hustle and bustle of a large and loud family.

Jay insists on the menu: Turkey, mashed potatoes with both brown and white gravy, squash and mushroom casserole, cranberry and pecan casserole, green beans with almonds, and white cake with white icing.

Jay leads us in Grace. "A-one, a-two, a-one, two, three…" he begins, counting off the cadence to our Grace.

"God is great, God is good," we all join him. "Let us thank Him for our food."

Knowing there is more, we do not eat, and Jay concludes, "Let's eat. Let's eat. Let's eat."

"Small bites!"

With that, he seizes a spoon and ladles a huge portion of mashed potatoes and brown gravy into his mouth. He is, as we said in North Carolina, "in hog heaven." His eyes light up as he eats his first bite of the holiday meal.

We smile broadly and raise our glasses for a toast. He swallows quickly, holds his glass high aloft, arm fully extended, and, before any of us can say a word, declares, "Cheers. Cheers to everyone!"

Christmas

Nearly a month passes. Jay remains in excellent humor, but he is eager for Christmas to come and go. It is the last major holiday of the year. Easter is far away. Jay thinks only about Christmas.

We fly to Chicago to be with Amy and her family. I ask for early boarding so Jay can be near the restroom, and the boarding agent, looking at Jay, agrees. Jay buckles himself into his seat. I sit next to him. Ann sits across the aisle.

"Peanuts, Coke," he says.

"Yes, Jay, soon. After we take off."

"Soon? Now?"

"Yes, soon," I reassure him.

"Bathroom," he declares.

Passengers are still boarding, but Jay will have his way. We stand up; the attendant stops the boarding while Jay and I go to the restroom. He enters and I stand outside; it is too small for both of us.

When he finishes, he opens the door. He has pulled his underpants up so high they stick out over his pants. I adjust his shirt, tucking it in. The stewardess allows boarding while Jay and I repair his attire. Jay is not at all perturbed; he and I do the "tuck in your shirt" routine at home and in the office, indeed, wherever we need to. Passengers are intent on boarding; some do not see us in the galley, others peer curiously at us, a father and fully grown son, doing what fathers do for their infant and toddler children.

Jay and I have our own meaning of normalcy; we are comfortable with it. It does not matter to us that others may not be. It has been that way for years; there is no changing our ways.

Returned to our seats, buckled in, and ready to take off, Jay and I restart the "peanuts and Coke" conversation. The engines start, the plane shivers, it taxis, it charges down the runway, and it is aloft. Jay mimics the engines, "hrmm, hrmm," and flaps his fingers. He is happy. Christmas is coming. So are peanuts and Coke. And much more, too.

PART IV

Death

So much of Jay's life is his leaving it on January 7, 2009. So much of his meaning comes from remembering him, from returning him to us, and in knowing that we will never be with him again in this life but that he never truly has left us.

Embedded in the following narrative is my candid revelation of the meaning of Jay's life for me and the effects Jay's death has had on me. I wrote spontaneously, in verse, a form I had never used before. I present my verses here, in the chronological order in which I wrote them.

There are some lessons here—

– about the necessity to be true to one's self;

– about the freedom from self that comes from offering unprotected vulnerability to others;

– about the arc of emotion and understanding that began

the day Jay died and, for this memoir, ends two years later, to the day;

– about the nature of writing—the writer's sense that he is alone in this world, a reader's sense that she is alone in this world, and their joint sense that they are not alone, that narrative and verse join them; and

– about the elegant mysteries of life, made known to us through symbols and the contexts and times in which they appear.

20
Closings

On the night of the day Jay dies, I retreat momentarily to my study and begin to write whatever comes to mind, trying to give words to my emotions. I surprise myself because the first word I write is "closings."

The word comes to me over and again. I record its many meanings. As a noun, it is a real estate or business transaction, the fence-enclosed yard around a church, an enclosing embrace of another person, an event such as the ending of a play or series of performances. As an adjective, it is a descriptor—to be a closer, a finisher; a geography—to be near. As a verb, it is a transitional action—the closing of a casket or the ending of a life; and with death, the beginning of new lives, an action—to close, and indeed, two verb uses—involuntarily, passively—to be closed out, and voluntary—actively: to close out, end.

There is closing for Jay's life, in one sense: Like a chapel within its close, Jay will always be with us, inside the protective fence of his family and my memory. But there is a closing in another sense: he is gone.

Prescience

There is a prescience about Jay's death that I do not understand.
A friend tells me: "You saw this coming, you intuited it, you sensed it
    months ago.
You and I talked about Jay and death in our last meeting before he died.
You have a sense of yourself, of what you need,
Of the world around you. Of a world beyond you."
She cannot explain it. Nor can I.

Preparation

I had begun to talk and write privately about life and death.
I had created the Jay Turnbull Fellowship to honor Jay.
Ann had concurred, but had asked, "Why now?"
I had purchased my cousin's paintings of my grandmother and father.
Ann had found them on-line, in a Baltimore auction house.

I had put into place all the action necessary for Jay's future:
The licensed corporation, JTSD, LLC: Jay Turnbull Self
    Determination;
The amendments to our Last Wills and Testaments and Trusts;
The meeting with the trustees in Baltimore, an agreement about a
    successor trustee;

The beginning of billing for Medicaid: freedom from the local agency.
Vocational Rehabilitation: approved.
Job coaching: charged to the state.
Plan of care: redone and re-filed.
Jay's court-required guardianship report: filed early.
Bureaucracy: satisfied.

Late in December, Jay had been to his regular dentist to fill his first
    cavity.
Tom and I were with him; he did not clamp down or flee in a panic.
He trusted Tom and me.

At Amy's, at Christmas, Jay was calm amidst the boisterousness of her
     home,
Tolerant of the busy-ness of the time and place.
He patted her young children gently, kissed them tenderly.

He had a single small outburst,
Enough to cause me to take him to his bed,
To lie down beside him, to touch him and calm him.

Tom and Laura had pledged to stay with Jay indefinitely,
But they had withheld their announcement.
They had knotted that loose end
Without my knowledge.
"We were going to tell you that we would stay with Jay indefinitely,"
They tell us on the horrid day he died.

Early in January, he had been to Michelle's for his haircut,
Not as short as Tom wanted, and just as long as I had wanted.
I was with him.
He let Michelle clean behind his ears and shampoo his scalp.
Those were acts of love. He loved being loved.

This was the haircut he would have at his death,
The "just right" haircut, not too short, nor too long:
Perfectly presentable for God.

Readiness

Ann and I had been in New Zealand in October.
We returned, energized by telling Jay's stories,
Buoyed by the families there.

We had learned that, for Maori,
The rubbing of noses was a gesture of peace.
Their gestures had been Jay's, Ann's, and mine.
At last we had learned their meaning.

Readiness was all.
Readiness for Jay:
His work was done, his teachings concluded.

It is as though he had judged us and found us to be worthy.
"OK, Dad and Mom, you got it right.
It's time for me to go."

A backward wave of his hand, as Kate tells us, signified,
"I've got it from here."

Symbolically, the pilot light in our fireplace went out
Early in the morning on the day Jay died.
We had expected light and heat.
We experienced the absence of each.

Readiness is all.
But I was not ready.

21

Last Days

Saturday and the "Brown Hotel"
(January 3, 2009)

The Saturday night before he dies, Jay goes to "the brown hotel" with
    Bryan.
He returns to our home on Sunday.
Walking toward me, his blue coat buttoned to his chin, his hood on,
His face nearly obscured, his gait slow, deliberate, splayed,
He is unhurried. This is a usual moment: hotel and then home.

He swings his suitcase against the walls of our home,
But such sweet bruising never bothered him,
For he is home, his room and family awaiting him.

All is as normal as it has ever been.
His mood is up, not over the top, just at its cusp.

Sunday, the Last Good-Night, and Unusualness (January 4, 2009)

Breakfast on Sunday is with Lauren Priest, his friend for five years,
Brunch with Marissa and John Clark and their children.
In top form, engaged, conversational, polite,
Surrounded by those who loved him,
Jay is in glory-land.

The last Sunday night:
He in his red pajamas, I in my matching set.
We eat well – steaks, his favorite meat,
Sprite to drink,
M & M chocolates for dessert,
Shared space on a green couch,
Mindlessly watching television.

"Jay, is it time to go to bed?" I ask.
He answers as always,
"Mom say prayers."

"No," I ask, "let me say prayers."
He accedes, reversing his usual routine, hinting at change.

He rises and leans over the couch to kiss Ann goodnight, nearly
    toppling onto her.
She raises herself, offers her face, stretches to receive his kiss.
They kiss, speak the dearest words, "I love you," each to the other.

And then he ambles to his room,
Following his usual indirect route, around the dining room table.

First, the entire prayer: "Our Father, who are in Heaven,
Hallowed be thy name…
For thine is the kingdom, and the power, and the glory forever."

And then the long remembrances:
"God bless Mom and Dad, Amy and Kate,
Rahul and Chip,
Laura and Tom,
TJ the dog,"

Then friends from his times in Massachusetts and North Carolina,
And at end, "God bless cereal and milk."

The people, and cereal and milk.
Kate had it right. It was the little joys of life that counted,
But only after the people.
They mattered to him, more than any other elements of his life.

Did Jay somehow sense that the long prayer was needed,
That it was to be his last prayer?

Was that last long prayer
A sign from the Divine through Jay to me?

The last usual acts, the last evening time,
Of our son-hood and father-hood
Are ceremonies of love, and always have been:

The last nosey-nosey in bed, the last kiss on his face,
The last soft rubbing of his hair,
The last tucking-in,
The final "Goodnight, I'll see you in the morning."

Monday and Usualness
(January 5, 2009)

The next morning, he awakes, soaking wet, not a rarity.
The customary shower, with more attention to his private areas.
He allows me to touch, to clean him.
Then the ordinary drying and dressing routine.
All is normal this Monday.

Breakfast at his usual café, preceded by his usual Grace:
"God bless bacon, eggs and pancakes."

Such usual-ness.
He eats with gusto. He is content, happy.

Then the drive to his home. He puts the visor up on both sides of the
     car,
Neatness and symmetry established, OCD manifest but calmed.
He hands me my briefcase and sends me on my way.

Thus I remit him to Tom, Laura, and Reagon, his morning care-giver,
Who found him dead on Wednesday.

Tuesday and the Black Shoes
(January 6, 2009)

I do not see Jay on Tuesday,
Only his black left shoe, visible between the partitions
In the bathroom we share.

He answers my question "How are you, son?" with two words,
"I'm fine."
He returns to work for the last time.

The Last Night

Sarah tells us: His last song-request on the last night of his life
Is "Swing Low, Sweet Chariot."

A chariot came to carry him home.
How did he know it was coming?

She refuses to end the music that way.
She and he sing one last song:
"You Are My Sunshine."

And all during the week after he dies
The sun shines gloriously.

22

The Last Day
(January 7, 2009)

"I'm Fine. Waffles"

Jay awakes happily and cheerfully.
It is his usual time, about 7:35.

"How are you, Jay," Tom asks.
Jay responds, "I'm fine."

"What do you want for breakfast, Jay," Tom asks.
Jay answers, "Waffles."

Jay begins his usual routine:
Out of bed, into the bathroom, sit on the toilet, shut the door.

Tom hears the clicking of latch on the door.
All is as normal as it could be.

Jay's last words, "fine" and "waffles."
Of course, all is well and food is coming.

The last words of his life are
Words of love and concern,
The usual words between best friends.

The Un-lifted Latch

Reagon arrives, spends a moment with Tom,
And walks to the bathroom to help Jay with his shower.

Tom tells us: "Whenever Reagon arrived, Jay would open the door,
We would hear the latch lift, and hear him greet her.
But we did not hear that this day."
His last sound on this earth: the latch shutting the door.

Discovery

Reagon discovers him.
She screams. Tom rushes in.

Jay is on the toilet, leaning to his right, against the wall.
His upper lip is blue.
Tom seeks a pulse in his neck, on his wrists.
No response, nothing there.
He lays Jay down, does CPR, mouth to mouth.

Reagon calls 911.
Tom, his efforts to revive Jay having failed,
Now calls me, "Rud, come fast, Jay is unconscious."
He calls Ann; she and Lois race to his home.
I arrive before them.
Police cars, ambulances, sirens, and flashing lights portend a macabre
    scene.

Chaos

On arriving, I see only his stomach.
Medics surround him, blocking my view.
He is pale yellow, or a sallow white.
I know: Jay is dead.

Ann arrives.
We sit, wait, and say not a word: we know.

There is chaos:
Medics, police, and coroners,
Shock paddles, drip lines, calls to the ER physician,
And Jay lying on the floor outside his bedroom door.

Releasing Life

Ann and I, solo in our own thoughts, think the same:
Jay will not still be alive but irreversibly comatose.
That is not who he is.

We turn to each other, our eyes and minds and hearts in union:
We speak the proclamation: We cannot bear it.
Let him go. This is the end.

Now the medics confess,
"We've done all we can."
Their efforts are unavailing.
As we knew they would be.

Such a pronouncement of death,
Delayed out of duty to try to bring life back,
Stated factually and with sorrow, announces,
It's over.

Acknowledgement

Ann and I turn to each other:
"We have lost him. Jay is dead."

It is a few minutes after 8.
Ann goes to him,
Rubbing his head, touching his hair, the only uncovered part of him.
She and I repeat the ritual.

We now pull down the sheet draping him.
Jay is blue, the intubation still in his mouth.
He is nearly unrecognizable,
Monstrously gagged by technology.

We say the Lord's Prayer.
Tom and Laura stand over us.
The police hover, for this is a crime scene.

Blue, Cold, and Gone

Our mortician friend Larry arrives from the funeral home.
Jay now lies on a gurney.
Larry removes the tubing;
The police will not allow us to do so, nor could I bear to touch him
     just then.
Larry covers him.
Our pastor Peter hurries to us from his church.

Peter prays for Jay and us, we say the Lord's Prayer, we hold hands.
I hear only words.
I cannot comprehend the prayer's meaning,
For there is but one meaning: Jay has left us.

I watch as Larry wheels Jay out, puts him into a white truck, and
Takes him from his home, never to return.

191

Demanding His Return

I go to the windows to watch as Jay is rolled away.
I scream, again and again, "I want my son back."
The rest of Jay's home is silent.
There would be no sound, only a void, but for my screams.

My agony does not stop. It repeats itself.
Over and over again.
It is the only life I have, the only antidote to shock.
Dozens of times. The same pain, the same wailing.

Ann weeps deeply, sometimes the loud cry of a bereft mother,
Sometimes the restrained cry of a brave mother,
Always, a mother in the deepest possible pain.
Her hurt can be touched, it is so palpable.

We hold each other.
We sob together, breathing in Jay's death as we did his life,
Together, in unison, as one.

A Decade in a Day

The rest of the day is one of shock.
I shake, I am cold, I shiver, I cover myself in coats.
It is shock. I've known it before.

We call our daughters:
"Jay has died."

Amy is wordless, her voice gagged by tears.
We hear her choke, and then we hear her sobs.

Kate screams: "No, he hasn't."
She repeats herself, denying this horrible news.

They arrive hours later.
Amy is loud in her grief.
Kate holds in, refusing to let go.

Each has her own way.
Each way is good and wholesome, like each of them.

Tom and Laura are stunned into silence.
I cannot imagine their grief.
They too have lost a son
For they said Jay was like a son,
They treated him as one,
And in doing so, they gave Jay and Ann and me and Amy and Kate
A great peacefulness, an absence from concern and worry.

I walk through the day, stooped, stunned, slowly, haltingly.
I have aged a decade in a day.

Surreal

Just hours after Jay leaves his home, we must plan the post-mortem
    ceremonies.
"It's all so surreal," Kate says.
We concur.
But it is all so very real.

Hardness

The planning is hard.
We do not agree entirely.
Each of us is strong,
Each has a way to memorialize him,
To comfort self and others.

There is hardness among us,
A rigidity, a rigor, born of love and shock.
Peter mediates.

I seek the Old Book of Common Prayer,
I want, need, the dirge, the grieving ceremonies
That I have read so often,
The paeans to God that I have marked in my Hymnal.
My family concurs.

Ann, Amy, and Kate seek a service that celebrates Jay's life,
Constructed around the music he loved.
I concur.

We find our compromises.

There is harmony at the end of the planning.
Of course there is harmony.
That was always Jay's way.

Sleep, Dream, and Recall

In half-wakefulness that night, memories come to me:
The people, food, and music Jay loved.
Mostly the music, the key to his soul.

"Kumbaya, My Lord."
"Michael, row your boat ashore, Alleluia," – the first sensible words he
        ever uttered to me.
"Prepare Ye the Way of the Lord" – St. Matthew's Gospel, set to music.
"Amazing Grace."
"Swing Low, Sweet Chariot."

All these, songs of faith.
And then songs of greeting,
John Denver: "Come, let me love you, come, love me again."

Again. As though I could do that physically.
The "Hello, JT," song,
Listing the people he loved and was loved by.

Ann's father had said,
"Jay doesn't pray for any SOB."

Either a person was within Jay's ambit of love-giving and receiving,
Or the person was unknown to Jay, a non-person.

Jay was too good for this world – so say some friends.
But that was not true: he was what the world needed,
And much of this world, and so many people,
Were good to Jay.

23
The Days After

Urns
(January 8, 2009)

On the first day after the day,
We all gather: Ann, Amy, Kate, Tom, and Laura.
Our purpose: to choose a casket: Done, too easily.

To chose the to-be-buried urn. Done, also too easily.
Likewise, four small urns, two for the Turnbulls,
Two for the Riffels.

A small urn will hold Jay; he cannot leave my home
So long as I have him there.

Preparation for the Public Ceremonies

Within hours of Jay's death, there is a torrent of flowers, food, emails,
       telephone calls,
Foretelling the hundreds who will come to say goodbye to Jay,
To mourn and celebrate with us,
To comfort – to strengthen – the remaining Turnbulls.

Colleagues arrive from our offices, nearby,
From their offices, miles away.
Jay is gathering the masses,
As he did in his lifetime.

Godparents arrive from North Carolina,
Ann's family from Georgia,
Friends from all points of the American compass,
Old and young, white and black, they assemble.

We cherish these moments with friends,
The handshakes and embraces,
They – not who – are what we remember during these ceremonies of
    death.

But of course we do,
For those were the contacts that Jay most loved and gave, most lovingly.

The Visitation
(January 9, 2009)

Ann, Amy, Kate, and I become hosts,
Greeting the hundred and more people as they enter the mortuary
    and re-enter our lives.
This role comes to me naturally,
For it was Jay's role as he greeted people at his home and ours.

Succor and strength come to me
From holding others, from comforting them, from assuring them,
From enclosing them and being enclosed by them
In embraces of sorrow and grief.

I become a teacher, guiding Jay's dearest friends to him.
I take their hands, we walk to Jay.
I ask, "May I touch him with you?"
And when they do not object, I take their hands in mine
And together we touch Jay's hair, for it is the most alive part of my
    son's corpse.

John Muller, a friend so dear he has become family,
Cannot bear to approach.
As John always does, he stands back, distant, observant.
"Come, John," I say, "we can come closer to Jay."
And so we do.

John and I embrace. And I confess what he has known:
"You are family to me." He understands:
He is like a son, but no one can be Jay.

The Funeral
(January 10, 2009)

Jay's friends fill the sanctuary, nearly 700 of them,
Overflowing it. No seat is unoccupied.

Brought together by Jay, people from all walks of life pay their respects.
Sarah Aldridge and her family – the black family who took care of
    Ann's father – are there.
They precede the Chancellor and Provost in the reception line.
The publisher of our paper had it right when he wrote that Jay was a
    cementing force.

But he is not there to greet them, not in his usual way.
He lies in the church's entry, his casket open.
He is clothed in his dress uniform: blazer, white shirt, red tie, gray
    trousers.

People enter, register in the books rested on lecterns.
Some pass him by, others come to him.
Again, I greet them, take some to see Jay, a few, to touch him.

Then, amidst the milling mourners,
Oblivious of them, contained wholly within myself,
I lift one of his rigor-mortised hands from the other,
Remove his wallet, with its $8, and his keychain, from his death-grip.

I try but cannot remove his watch and ring.
A funeral assistant removes them
And hands them to me.

These are Jay's artifacts.
I place them into my briefcase.

From it I withdraw scissors.
I clip two locks of his hair, recoverable, impermeable body parts for
    the future.
I comb his hair, repairing it,
Making him more the man he was,
Knowing he will never be that man, my son, again.

Our pastor Peter calls me to a small communion of the sorrowful,
Gathered in an anteroom adjacent to the sanctuary.

Ann introduces each of us to the other,
We join hands and pray.

It is time for us to come to Jay for the last time, to this Jay, to this
    remainder.
There are tears, embraces, closings.

Ann bends to him, kisses him, talks to him,
Words none of us hears. It is her private moment.
She has been his true mother.

Amy, then Kate, kneel beside his coffin, each alone,
Speak their adieus,
Seeking their separate peace, even as he now has his.

I come to him, rub his hair, lay my hands on his face,
Rub his nose with mine, and kiss his lips. I can make no noise.
It is as though I too were dead inside, though I am all too alive
With grief and pain.

There is now a closing:
The lowering of the casket's lid,
The locking of the top to bottom,
A permanent sealing.
The wooden tomb forbids any further touching.

The service glorifies God and Jay.
Sarah sings his favorite songs,
Urging the sanctuary-filling mourners to join her, affirming the joy of
        Jay's life.
"Hello, J.T., Hello, J.T., Hello, J.T., How are you today?" she sings.
He cannot answer. We know an answer: He is dead.
But we do not know how his spirit is.

Kate eulogizes Jay. She is his poet, for all she says and does
Brings sorrow and laughter, the perfect combination for Jay.
Two colleagues declare Jay's dignity and worth.

Peter speaks a pastor's comfort.
He knows Jay and captures him and our family perfectly.

I weep uncontrollably, not caring about – not being able to care about –
Any one except Jay, Ann, Amy, and Kate.
I cannot staunch my tears, nor do I try.

I am honest with my family and myself,
And with the other mourners:
This is my son, whom I have lost.

You see my love for him in the grief that wracks me,
You hear it in my wailing.

I silently ask, please let me have him back.
And yet I do so speed him away,
For he has lived magnificently and died mercifully.

The Lord's Prayer now means more than it ever did.
I hear Jay – not myself, for I cannot mouth a single word,
Not the mourners, for I am wholly within myself – speaking:
"Give us this day our daily bread," our ration of mercy and comfort.
"And forgive us our trespasses,"
As we know we have not done all we might have done for Jay.

"Thy will be done, on earth as it is in Heaven."
Jay is the Lord's gift to us.
Kate eulogized that Jay always on loan to us,
An angel walking the streets of Lawrence.
Jay's mission has been accomplished.
And so he was raised to God, brought home again.

"For thine is the Power," Jay emphasizing the Power,
Evidencing that he was indeed one of the Power-ful.
"And the glory."
Jay gloried in the Spirit.

I follow him and my family out of the sanctuary.
I have no shame in my tears, in my grief.
I repeat out-loud the obvious, "This is so hard, so hard."

Family and friends gather in a large meeting room,
Remember Jay with joy, their counter-balance to our sorrow.

I look around, nearly expecting to see Jay
Gulping lemonade,
Ingesting a cookie in one large bite.

I imagine helping him navigate the throng,
Aiding others to take his handshake,
Allowing him to give them his unique self.
But Jay is not there.

I return to his casket, and touch it where it covers his head.
"Travel well, JT, old boy."
I correct myself, as Jay would have corrected me:
"Old man!"

We take Jay out of the church,
I hold the door open, fearful of nicking his casket,
Thinking, it soon will be dust, and he will be ashes.

I remove my Turnbull Dress Tartan scarf,
Tie it to the casket, insist it be taken with him,
That it be part of him.
I had done the same when Mother died:
Laying Turnbull kilts on her coffin, I bid her a last farewell.

Celebration
(January 10, 2009)

At the celebration of his life that night,
More than 100 of Jay's family and friends gather for dinner.

Della coaxes us into singing one of Jay's favored songs.
It is John Denver's ode to his lover, "Annie's Song."
For 20 years, it was the coda to his music therapy sessions,
And to the many parties he hosted at his home.

His friends now sing it, raising their voices to him, celebrating his life.
"Come, let me love you, come, love me again," they sing.

They ask for his return, for the impossible.
He has asked them to come to him, to let him love them, and they
    have gone to him.
Now, they ask the same, futile in their request.
I weep. Jay is not there to sing with us.

Ann has a different closing in mind – not "Annie's Song," but another.
She tells these witnesses to Jay's life,
"We usually closed all of our parties with that song.
"But tonight, because we will never be able to sing it again with Jay,
"Let's close with another song, one to honor his life.
"At the tables where you are sitting is a small candle for each of you.
"Please light the candle. Hold it aloft. And join me in singing about Jay.
"The song is, 'This Little Light of Mine, I'm Going to Let It Shine.'"

She lights a candle, Jay's friends light theirs.
All hold their candles aloft, the lights dim,
And we all sing, "This little light of mine."
Jay's picture is projected onto a screen.
His image is smiling as we are weeping.

The Burial
(January 12, 2009)

The burial, two days later, is somber and brief.
Jay's ashes are in urns, one large one and five miniatures.

Peter says a prayer.
I ask, "May I say a few words."
My wish granted, my voice trembles.

I recite the first verse of "Victory."
"The strife is o'er, the battle done,
The victory of life is won."
I need no hymnal. I know "Victory" by heart.

"The three long days of death are done,
"All glory to the risen Son."
I weep at the "Alleluia," closing this last ceremony.

The sun has shone on us each of these days.
From Wednesday to Sunday, the Kansas sky has been clear and blue.
The moon has been as full as it will be for the next 12 months.

Our friend Peggy has told us a Greek legend:
Angels and risen spirits dance on the moon.
Jay now dances with the angels,
Again offering us the light of his life.

PART V

Grief, God, and Gratitude

24
The Days Subsequent
(January 12 and thereafter, 2009)

And now begins a newness so unwelcome.

Being Whole

Amy affirms, "Jay was a whole person."
Kate elaborates, To be whole is to have all parts of life,
The imperfections coupled with the perfections,
With acceptance of that wholeness by one's self and by others.

Jay accepted himself as a whole person,
And so did so many others.
Jay taught about whole-ness,
For his whole-ness
Consisted of unconditionally loving himself and others,
Of not passing judgments based on traits or status,
Of creating community – the shared togetherness –
That typified his life.
He has taught us about being whole.

Going Through the Motions

At night, in our home, we expect Jay in his usual places in our home,
But we do not enter his room, knowing he is not there.
Each of us remembers this past Sunday, seven days ago,
The first day of our week of utter newness.

Amy and Kate return to their homes.
Ann and I now go through the motions of this post-mortem life.
We return to work.

She, battling tears as she works, fails.
They come, her stoicism overcome.
She cannot utterly dike them.

Why is it so necessary to do the ordinary
After the occasion of the extra-ordinary?
I know the answer:
Because doing the ordinary is an antidote to the extraordinary.

The ceremonies of death are ended.
The business of accommodating to death begins.

The reversion to normalcy is so abnormal, so out of line, deviant.
I am angry, and, with guilt, relieved that I can return.

And yet I want the extraordinary back again:
My son, the far-from-ordinary man.

Reading Our Eulogies
(January 18, 2009)

We avoid church on the Sunday after burying Jay.
I go to my office and spend hours responding to mail about Jay.
Each letter tells the same story.

Jay inspired us.
He mattered to us, to our world.
You, his parents, were his parable-tellers,
Speakers to our hearts.

Kate telephones and interprets the letters for Ann and me:
"You are reading your own eulogies."

Snowflakes

Only one letter says anything about our research or advocacy,
Research on how to live a life of great expectations and unusual dignity,
Advocacy so that such a life would obtain.

Like snowflakes, each letter is unique, slightly different than any other.
Like an avalanche, they bury us
Yet give us a passage to breathe.

Within this avalanche, we inhale in the writers' words,
And we exhale Jay.

To breathe him out is to still give life to him,
Though his ashes lie silent.
To give life to him – that is the letters' effect.

The Ability to Be, Not to Do

Jay was so limited yet so abundantly gifted,
An infant written off by physicians and some family,
Compulsorily abandoned to the care of strangers,
And then centered in a community
Because, in his way, he created community.

Jay's gifts were not his ability to do,
But his ability to be,
Simply to say
"Come, let me love you,
Come, love me again."

Or, "I get by with a little help from my friends."
Or, "Mine eyes have seen the glory of the coming of the Lord."
Or, "Kumbaya, my Lord, come to me."

So many songs. Jay knew them all.
All were about largesse of the spirit
And gifts of self.
What more is there to give
Except Jay?

The Jay-Space

Having avoided any place where Jay had worked,
I must sometime confront his office, and I do.

There is his chair, its arms worn, its back and seat depressed by his body.
There is the shredding machine, inanimately waiting for him to feed it.
There are the photographs of his job coaches.
They embrace him
And give him cause to smile his largest smiles.

Laura's sign still is on the wall next to Jay's desk,
Posted 8½ years earlier.
"If JT can't do it, no one can."
It proclaims her affirmation of his ability,
Her faith in him.

There is his calendar, each day waiting to be crossed off in green ink.
The last day is crossed off: Tuesday, January 6.
It has been two weeks since he left work, never to return.
His name-plate is still on the office door.
Closings elude us.
The physical world has not changed,
We have not caused it to change.

We hold fast to it, for the spiritual is far too much with us.
And yet, in holding to the physical world,
To the detritus of his work,
We deny his death.

I cannot bear the openness of his work station.
It has not changed at all, it awaits him in vain.

I return to my office, cursing, angry.
And then I cry again – hard, long, sobs.

Ann comes to touch me.
She gives comfort.
But I still want that little touch of Jay.
"I want him back," I wail.
"I want my son back."

The Best Way to Die
(week of January 26, 2009)

Ann and I meet my newly appointed cardiologist.
Describe Jay's medical history, his death,
And hear the doctor's lecture about a heart's physiology.

His last words confirm our beliefs, our deepest hopes:
Ventricular fibrillation – instant arrest of the heart, instant non-
    existence.

No warning. No pain. Nothing. Just instant death.
The best way to die, bar none.

Mercy and a Gift

Death was merciful.

Ann and I are relieved,
For Jay's sake and ours.
He has no more worries,
No more reasons for explosions and depressions.

Guiltily, I sense relief.
Yet Margaret Ann Schwartzburg's words console me:
"Job well done, Rud.
"Jay did not want you to worry any more, to work any more.
"His death was his gift to you."

Death as a gift. The paradox is too great.
And yet there is truth here.
Death was merciful to him, for he did not suffer.

And to us, for we did not have the duty of care
That would have attended him and us
Had he lived longer and become ancient or died otherwise.

There is surcease from work and worry.
Doubt visits me:
Why do I feel so conflicted, why such convoluted feelings?

25
Frozen and Shocked
(January 12-31, 2009)

Frozen

Ann declares, "We are frozen in time."
No more Jay to teach us; no future with him.
Only the past. We are fossilized.

The Jay-embrace is not to be. Never again.
Scent will dissipate; embraces will elude;
Some closings will occur,
But not soon the one in our hearts:
The wound is agape.

Now, fearless of Jay's future, we are nearly rootless:
We no longer must care for our man-child.
We have lost our norm.

No new life with Jay to experience,
No new stories to tell.
We question our legitimacy: parents no longer, just professionals.
Of course, that is not true,
But, of course, it is.

Shocked and Occluded

Ann and I have fuzzy minds.
We cannot concentrate easily.
We become more forgetful.
Lists accompany us wherever we go.

"Shock," I say to her.
"We are still in shock."

Not the kind that I have felt while waiting for surgeons
After wounds and organ failures.
Not the kind I felt during the week of death and ceremonies:
That shaking, that cold, those unusually antic moods,
Those uninterrupted tears.

This shock is different. It is subtle and sneaky.
It blurs our life. What has been transparent, easily seen,
The substance of each day of our earlier lives,
Is now occluded, difficult to discern.
We want clarity. We want Jay himself, not memories of him.

26
Gifts
(January 12-31, 2009)

The Gift

I often told my students:
We must give our children away.
We must give Jay to his community.
And so we did, Ann, Amy, Kate and I.

Here, we said, offering him to our friends, students, communities:
Here is Jay. He belongs to us but you too may have him.
Please accept him, please take him.
He needs you. We need you.
You need him.

We gave people a chance to be part of his life.
If they responded, as they often did, then Jay belonged,
And how he belonged!

Our Best Professor

Ann and I were but instruments for Jay and his mission.
We all were only that, simply the means to his life.
Jay lead us, guided us, demanded of us,
Stubbornly refused any life but the one he wanted.

Yes, he was our best professor,
But he never gave us a course
For this final examination,
Except the one that Kate described,
The lesson about loving and living as Jay did.

He was more than our professor.
He was, in his way, a creator,
A person come to us to save us,
To imbue our lives with meaningfulness,
To teach us and cause us to teach.

His teaching was purposeful:
Follow me, he said, and you and I will find life together.
The enviable life, Ann and I have called it.

27
Beyond the Immediacy
(January 22-31)

Resurrection (January 22, 2009)

Thursday, two weeks and a day since Jay died,
Just under two since we buried him,
I go to his grave.

A modest plastic marker informs:
"Jay Turnbull, 1967–2009."
The soil has been poured over him,
The sod replaced.

The cavities between the newly placed sod and the old are wide.
I could easily lift the sod, dig the soil,
Reach down, lift his urn, hold him again.
Resurrection.

I do nothing except shake my fist in anger and cry.
He has been resurrected already.

His remains remain: I do not disturb them.
But he also remains,
As much inside me as inside the buried urn.

Sorrow's Companion

I wait at Michelle's studio to have my hair cut.
On the wall in her studio, three memories hang:
A photograph of Jay and me, arms around each other, laughing,
A photograph of Jay at the beach, sitting cross-legged on the sand,
    content,
Both taken three or four years ago.
Below them, Kate's eulogy.

My heart quickens, I hear it work, I feel it pound.
Grief takes its physical toll,
And tears return.

Michelle reaches down to me, seated in a chair,
Pulls my head to her breast, and lets me wet her.
She too loved Jay, and now her tears moisten my head.

Sorrow needs a companion
And finds one in another person.

Apparitions
(January 2–February 7, 2009)

Death surprised us. It came suddenly, massively, mercifully.
Jay is gone.
Never and forever: the two cruelest words.
Never to be held again. Forever absent.

Except in our minds and hearts.
And then – as suddenly as Jay died –
He returns.

Fine

In my half-sleep, Jay appears,
On this, the 14th day after he died,
Reprising the visit he paid the day after he died.

He is dressed in a white shirt, red tie, and blue blazer:
His dress uniform.
His face is nearly indiscernible,
Nearly blank.

He has an aura of peacefulness,
Of being alive and pacific, calm.
His apparition assures me.
I nearly hear his familiar, dismissive refrain:
"I'm fine, just fine."

He signals contentment by a wave of his hand,
Wanting to be left alone in death, as in life,
Seeming to say, "Let me rest in peace."

Peace

This, the 15th day after Jay died, begins with signs:
Jay appears to me as I awake.
He is dressed as if at a party:
White shirt, red tie, blue blazer –
His uniform for an occasion of laughter and delight.
And his go-to-the-grave garb, as well.

His apparition is content.
It shows neither delight, nor fear, nor anger.
There are only contentment, harmony, and peace.

I see them in his apparition.
Truly see them. Not just want to see them,
But see them.

Inseparable

Nearly a month after Jay died, he revisits me in my narcotic sleep.
He is younger by 10-15 years.

I reach out to him, seeking his consent
To kiss him on both cheeks.
He assents, and I hug him,
But he keeps a short distance between himself and me,
As he always did except when he was sad.
Now, he is peaceful, content, harmonious.

That same night,
Ann dreams that she and Jay are walking, arms locked.
She urges him to walk more quickly but he will not.
He had his own pace in life, and we honored it, sometimes reluctantly.

The next night, Jay re-appears to me,
This time as a child, holding me, his curls brushing my face.

He is not an apparition while I am awake and working.
It is only afterwards, when my world stops, that he enters into it.
We are inseparable.

Never Again

Some few days later, Jay comes to me early in the morning.
He puts his two blue pillows on my bed, near my face, where they
 belong,
At the head of the bed.

I hear him speak to me the words I often spoke to him,
"Get up, Dad, put your feet on the floor."

There is – but never will be again – the get-up routine.
There is – but never will be again – the good-night one,
His scrunching up the pillows under his head,
My telling him, "Scoot down," and trying to rearrange them
So he could breathe more easily.

No touching, no lying down together, no calming by embracing,
No sight of him sitting in a chair or on a toilet.

The bathroom:
A place for morning expectations,
And a place for Death.

Anchored in the Past, Healing for Today
(January 28, 2009)

Three weeks after Death came,
Amy and Kate return; Ann and I meet them at Jay's home.
They have been sitting in his room.
They emerge, red-faced, tear-streaked.

They have grieved in his bedroom,
Almost in his presence, for his smell is still there.
We embrace, closing into one the four survivors of the fifth one.

Cataloguing the Past
(January 28, 2009)

There is healing in being in Jay's home that day,
Gleaning through the past, cleansing the present by abandoning the
    superfluous.
We spend three days anchored in the past, in the artifacts,
    photographs, and memories.

Amy and Kate miss the concreteness, the palpability of Jay's physical
    presence.
They want to hold him, hear him, smell him, hear him.
Their senses ache for him.

At our home, not his, we sort and catalogue photographs.
These open his life to us again.

We travel through the past.
Amy and Kate pour over the albums and artifacts I have kept.
They giggle and exclaim, their memories jarringly happy.

Detritus
(January 29, 2009)

On the second day of this Jay-less reunion,
In Jay's home,
I empty the drawers in his bathroom,
The combs and brushes, the toothpaste and toothbrushes,
Soaps and deodorants.

All those keeping-clean tools,
Evidence of the care-giving, must be jettisoned.
Useless to others, particular for him and him alone.
They must go. He went away. So, too, they must go.
They are the detritus of his life.

Empty Sleeves
(January 29, 2009)

In time, we have no more boxes to haul up or away.
But there remain his closets.
I open them, his hall closet first.
His blue coat, the one he wore on his last weekend visit to me,
Hangs askew.
His hat, scarf, and gloves rest on the shelf above his coat,
Lifeless.

We look at the clothes in his closet, awaiting him,
Pants folded, shoes aligned, shirt-sleeves empty.

His clothes are tangible, sensuous remembrances of him.
We see, smell, nearly hear and taste him.
He nearly returns to us.
Nearly. But of course, not at all.

Jay's physicality is so present, so acute.
This room was his – not a decoration in it,
Jay, a minimalist, a monk, cutting life to the core in his own space,
Knowing – better, sensing – that much is superfluous.

Nothing teaches more about finality
Than the shirt sleeves.
They beg to be brought to life, to have a physical occupant.

The Dissipating Scent
(January 29, 2009)

We absorb his impermanent scent,
Bag the clothes he would have worn the day he died,
Remove his pillows, sheets, and bed-spread,
Hold them to us, breathe in his essence.

Kate opens the drawers to his dresser,
Withdraws his pajamas, smells them, and sobs.
She stands alone, his clothes to her face,
Seeking his essence, a scent in lieu of a touch or voice.

Frozen and Naked
(January 29, 2009)

Time freezes here and now.
Just as his room, his own special place, is naked of all but the essentials,
So too are we.

Our emotions bare themselves.
Kate leaves and weeps violently in the spare bedroom,
Staring into his other closet.

Amy sits in his chair,
Soaked in tears,
Almost breathless, soundless.

The common sorrow brings us together.
We hold each other, four lonely family survivors.

Curls
(January 29, 2009)

That night, at our home, we return to our past.
I bring an envelope to the dining room table, convene my daughters
    and wife.
I open it, and from it fall locks of Jay's hair, from his first haircut.
Their golden colors have lost their gleam, their shine.
But the curls are there, twisting into a cornucopia of memories.

We touch them gently, as if we were touching him as a baby,
Lovingly, as though he were still alive.
And then we replace them, putting them into the paper envelope
That now substitutes for the wooden coffin.

His baby and death curls are preserved.
They are the residue, the last physical part of him,
The golden hair that mimed an angel's.
The rest is dust, resting in a tiny urn in his room.

Safe-keeping them safe-keeps Jay.
It is our way of continuing to care for him,
Not in the literal sense of caring about him, being concerning for him,
But literally having hands-on care.

Captured on Film
(January 29, 2009)

Videos reprise the photographs we have viewed,
But they make his him livelier, his life more vivid:

The *Charles Kuralt* show, with Jay saying prayers, a grace he repeated
    daily thereafter.
Amy and Kate sparkle, Ann and I comment and teach an unseen
    audience.
We are all so young. The year, 1983.
The last frame captures Jay dancing with Amy and Kate and then with
    Ann and me:
The dance of life, the joy of music.

That video presages another video, one of Jay at his office party.
Twenty years have passed.
But Jay is the same: still dancing, cute, flirtatious, energized, smiling,
    laughing.
He is in his element: music plays, a dance partner comes forward,
And Jay becomes the embodiment of liveliness, of life itself.

After Dad Dies
(January 29, 2009)

The next video has special portent,
In it, I model how to say goodnight to Jay
So that others would know his and my routine
And do as we do, after I die.
But Jay died first.

He and I play the "blanket game,"
Our heads together under the blanket I placed over my head,
Making our own special sounds, the "hunga-hunga" pig-grunt sounds,
Laughing and dancing before he lies down.

Then he goes to his bed, pulls up his covers, and I kneel beside him.
"Our Father," we intone. The full Lord's Prayer. Emphasis on "the
    Power."
And then the long recitation of called names.

Next, rubbing our noses together, our own Maori greeting of peace.
Then the goodnight kisses, left cheek, right cheek, forehead, nose, mouth.
Lights out.
"Goodnight, T-man. I love you."
"Good night, Dad. I love you, too."

The tapes evidence his and our lives.
We watch him and us, alive in so many of our Turnbull ways.

Jay has not changed over the last 20 years.
His smile, his sparkling eyes, his voice:
What he was at 21, he was at 41,
Just larger in the waist, a bit of gray speckling his hair.

Amy sobs, Kate maintains her pained silence,
Ann and I weep.

This is the common sorrow again, the time replayed in his room,

The clock and all time returned to January 7 and the days thereafter.

Our ceremony, our tribute to Jay,
Our memories of him and us,
Teaches that family is all, nothing else matters.

This is a moment of exquisite love,
A binding of five souls and four people,
For one person is gone,
Present only in the magnetic tapes we have watched,
Or in the spirit. That's it: Jay's spirit remains with us.

Nothing, but Everything, Changed

It is easy to bring back the memories, decades of them.
Nothing changed –
Until January 7.
There is such joy in the memories,
And such pain.
Sharpness – acuity – like we have not known since early January,
Exhausts us.

We stagger to bed,
Depleted, wholly voided,
And grieve ourselves to sleep.

Possessions and Possessing

The next day, Amy and Kate are speechless, silent, inward-bound.
They decline to talk about Jay.
They admonish us: "We have done too much too quickly."

They plead: "Give us time to be alone, to have our own ways these days."
They take Ann's car and drive away, destination unknown.
They go to Jay's home and return,

Arms full of artifacts, desired possessions held close to their hearts.

Shirts, hats, scarves, hand-painted picture frames leave Lawrence,
Bound for Chicago and New York.

Jay's yellow blanket – the one he treasured so – has been found,
And now is returned to us, kept safe in the bottom drawer of his chest
    in our home.
Next to it, Jay's red and white striped bathrobe, and the urn.
They join the artifacts from his funeral.

To possess his possessions is to possess him,
As much of him as we can.

28
Peaceful Symbols
(February, 2009)

Butterflies in Winter
(February 1, 2009)

We four lonely survivors – Ann, Amy, Kate, and I –
Conclude our purging and cataloging of Jay's past.
It is time for my daughters to leave.

But first, a trip to a store, to buy coffee.
There, Ann sees a stained-glass butterfly.
It has the black and blue wings of the one that came to Kate
The day we brought her home after she was born,
The same colors as of those my alma mater's teams.

The butterflies of Kate's first days had visited Ann's mother
When she was laid down in her Georgian grave.
They came, too, to Ann's father,
Buried 30 years later, to the day, in the same red-clay plot.

We see on the stained-glass two initials.
From one side, they are JT.
From the other, TJ.

Our son, JT.
His dog, TJ.

Ann and my daughters weep.
I, astonished at the symbol, am unable to do so.

Egg-Rolls, Chinese Cookies, and Friendship (February 1, 2009)

Later that day, I alone visit Jay's grave.
The marker is still there.
I remove the artificial flowers the wind has blown onto his grave from
    others.
His marker now reveals an egg-roll and a fortune cookie.
An old friend has been there,
His weekly lunch-mate.

Tributes take many forms, the most familiar being the best –
Food that Jay loved, given by a man
Who loved him and was loved in return.

Rather than tears and anger,
Such as I felt on my previous visit to Jay's grave,
I now own a not-yet familiar, all-too-new sense,
A sense of impeding difference in understanding,
Of variety in emotional response.

29

Honoring and Retrieving Jay
(January and February 8-14, 2009)

Honoring Jay in His Home

Tom and Laura, in a house that is no longer full of his life,
Avoid his room
Where normalcy awaited before Death intervened.

It is as though they know about sacred places,
About not disturbing them and the person they housed.

They explain why they were dedicated indefinitely:
"Jay was a member of our family."

One does not leave a family member.
That person leaves the family, as Jay left both families,
And all those others not related to each other except through him.

Retrieving Jay

Tom, Laura, and I go to the basement.
For the first time ever,
I open the drawers to the file cabinets
And admit them to his past.

The records begin at Johns Hopkins Hospital,
And end the month he died.

I vow to archive these records.
They tell about the struggles,
They capture the hardness
And make more glorious
His truly wonderful years.

Darkness and light.
Those are the hues of these records,
Their voided-ness and their luminosity.
It has not been easy, this living with Jay,
But it has been a cinch,
Compared to this living with his dying.

30
Wanting
(January, 2009 and thereafter)

Gestures

I want Jay back,
To have him fill that office openness where he once worked,
To have him plug the hole in my life,
To have him continue to be the source of stories,
The stories that people, known and unknown to me,
Remember with vigor:
"Stories about Jay changed my life."

My hungers are for his presence, his life, again,
And for its significance,
And for what would have been yet more significance.

I yearn for him in yet other ways, in the Jay-Dad ways
That have nothing to do with stories and meaning,
And everything to do with the gestures of love:

His handshake when he delivered my mail,
His clumsy emptying of the recycling box in my office,
His balled up and useless paper towel to dry his hands in the bathroom.

In elevators, I would turn his hat sideways, or put it onto my head.
He would always return it to its proper jaunt, on his head.
We would rub noses when no one else was with us.

When others entered, he would not step aside but reach to shake their
    hands.
I would introduce them,
"I want you to meet my son, JT,"
Watch them fumble to return his special handshake, learned from Pat
    and Corey,
And then teach them to accept him as he is,
As he offers himself to them.

He and I had our secret touches, our common gestures of love.
He modified me, insisting I put away my button-down-ness,
And enjoy his way of being in this world.
I complied and lived more richly than I ever could have lived otherwise.

For months after he dies, I am aware that a part of me is gone,
Not just one part, but many parts – the oh, so very physical.

He does not recede, but is purely absent.
Memories of him fill me, but he, the physical self, retreats.

The memories bring him back.
The paradox is undeniable and peculiar:
I want the "nearer" part of it, but even as I seek it by writing about him,
He – the incorporated Jay – takes his distance of me.

Denying
(January 21, 2009)

In class, the first of the semester, just days after Jay dies,
I do not mention Jay,
I do not draw my students' attention to the Preface of my book
Describing his early and then final years.

I deny his having lived,
For if I had signified his life,
The tears and anger would have returned,
Disabling me from teaching.

It is not possible to love in the touching-him way.
We must love his spirit.
How shall I teach that?

Even the places we shared with him –
His bedroom in our home and in his,
His office – remind us of him.

They are open, vacant,
He is dead, gone.
I cannot deny his death,
Nor yet affirm his life.

Acknowledging Jay
(March 10, 2009)

Nine weeks after Jay dies,
I mention him in class, for the first time.
Acknowledging his death, saying, for the first time,
That he will not be exemplar of my arguments, of my professing.
The rawness is too great, I admit.
I ask, "Please indulge me."

There is a moment of silence, of embarrassment,
A mute tribute to Jay.

31
Fusion
(February and March, 2009)

Peace, the Absence of Distress

Late in February,
Some sense of completion enters me.
I seek to reject it, to abolish the sense of closing.

But that sense stays, and, with it, comes a faux, partial peace.
Not genuine peace, not full peace,
But at least the absence of shock, grief, and deep at-the-core sorrow.

Peace: the absence of distress,
At least at some times.

At other times, there is simply Resignation.
Disbelief, yes. Anger, yes. Grief, yes. Mourning, yes. Sorrow, yes.
These old friends are still with me.
They have displaced Shock.

But Peace, or perhaps her cousin Resignation, or perhaps both
Have taken their places alongside them
And seem to be moving them aside.

Ann sees it in me, welcomes it, as I sometimes do.
I must now radically accept
That life entails death.

The Origins of Peace

Where is Peace's source?
Is it in my faith in the resurrection of the spirit?
In my obligatory bow to the duties that attend the business of death?
In my daughters' presence?
In Ann's strength to persevere?
In the physician's reassurance about the manner of death?
In the symbols we find – the stained glass portraying butterflies and
    initialed JT,
In the egg-roll and cookie laid at his grave?
In the compassion of a therapist, now a dear friend?
In the faith of a pastor, also a soul-intimate friend?
Yes, I answer to all questions.
Peace has multiple sources.

Perhaps, too, she comes to me in the company of Resignation,
The sense that there is nothing I can do but accept.

To accept, however, is nearly to say, "Jay's death is not objectionable."
I cannot say that. It is most objectionable, most horrible.

But it is unchangeable, immutable, complete.
And I must submit to it.

I still yearn for the massive tears and the pain.
I also know they will come, unexpectedly.
I know they will frequent me less often.
They are becoming strangers.

It is now time, I tell myself, to learn how to celebrate Jay's life.
To be authentic about that education and its end point – celebration.
Let the learning begin, I plead.
But learning is hard work, and slow to mature.

Fusion

There seems to be an integrity now,
A fusion of senses and feelings,
A wholeness,
A family of sisters.

Shock, Disbelief, Anger,
Grief, Mourning, Sorrow,
Now Peace and Resignation,
Love and Faith
Fuse with each other.

No other event, no other passage,
So sharpens these sisters' effects as Death,
So accentuates Love as Death.

The Good Pain

I still seek the deep hurt.
It comes now, less often,
So I stimulate it.

I hold his wallet and money, his key chain and ring.
I read Kate's eulogy.
I sob again, unable and unwilling to control myself.
It is good – it is healing – to let go.

Paradoxes

Time and again, I nearly drown in the paradoxes:
Doing the ordinary for the extraordinary man,
Being grateful about Death but being angry,
Denying but accepting,
Accepting the relief
While still feeling the grief.

32

Openness
(February and March, 2009)

Again

John Denver's verse haunts me:
"Come, let me love you, let me lie down beside you."

Jay's last outburst, Christmas, was at Amy's.
We lay down beside each other.

"Come, let me love you, come, love me again."
Again.

The words anticipate re-visitations, repetitions.
They carry hope,
And despair, for there is no "again" with Jay.

To lose the Alpha,
Requires us to confront the Omega.

Openness

In this cold winter of 2009, I revisit the discourses I had with myself in
    2007 and 2008:
The exploration of my intermittent angry blues.

In yesterdays of darkness and depression, in those two years before
    Jay died,
I thought about a vacuum, about the emptiness of myself.
Now, after Death, I reprise the idea of a vacuum,
About emptiness, about Death sucking Life away.

A friend asks me to think about openness.
That word is less threatening than vacuum;
It suggests that I yet have power to be potent, not passive.
But potent to what end? That is the question.

Emptiness

Empty.
It is a nasty word.
So too "never" and "forever."
These are cruel words.

Not that I fear I will be empty forever
And never be full.

It is just that, now, feelings and thoughts
Fail to fill the void, the vacuum, the openness.

Indeed, they enlarge it.
They force me to account for their cause:
Jay's death, his never-more-ness in the ways I once knew and had him,
His forever-gone-ness.

33
Remembering
(Winter and Spring, 2009)

Dismemberment

Death dismembers.
It takes away part of us.
And only memory can put back what is forever gone,
And even memory fails to satisfy wholly,
For the physical being – the Jay whom I held and kissed and cleaned
and comforted –
Is unobtainable.

All of these feelings and thoughts
And all the memories – only a portion of Jay's life,
For much more of it remains to be recalled –
Fail to fill the emptiness that has become part of me,
That threatens to be me.

Not Just of Semen Alone

Jay was a member of my body.
There was, with him, a physical intimacy
Born not just of semen alone,
But of 41 years of being his intimate care-giver.

Jay's death dismembers.
It is not an amputation, which deprives a person of a limb,
But a disemboweling, taking away a vital organ
But leaving me still alive.

Made One, Together

To remember is to bring back again, in one's mind,
The person remembered,
To re-call, as in re-gathering the person around one's self,
To re-member, as in making the person a member of one's life again.

To bring Jay back is to remember him,
As in re-membering, re-incorporating him.

To incorporate is to
To create a union,
A one-ness.

Death dis-members, and memory re-members.
Taken away, Jay returns through my mind.

It is not enough. I want his touch, his body, his smell, his voice.
I want him, and Death denies me.
Is it not right to be angry, so angry?

There is no way around it – this thing called living past Jay's death –
    but to go through it.
To go through it, to journey deeply into it, to embrace it, for to do that
Is to embrace Jay and his living-ness and meaning,
And my own as well.

Haunted

I am haunted by being in the spaces and times we occupied together.
We have walked down the hallways of the building where we work,
Jay strutting his quick-march,
I in close-march behind him, my hands on his hips.

We were not just of the same body and blood.
He was more than my manly consequence.

For 41 years, we were father-son, man and man-child,
Doing unusual small kinds of living
Because ordinary big living was not for him.

Bulls and Buttons

I dream:
In our home, one chandelier falls and breaks one of my bulls-head
    statues.
All that remain are four bulls' heads, not five.

I try to sleep and nap.
Involuntarily, I hear
"Somewhere, over the rainbow, way up high … "

I cry deeply.
I welcome the pain and fears. I want the hurt.

I awake, shower, dress.
I am buttoning my left back pocket.
Jay comes to me, telling me, as he always did, "Button,"
And pointing to both buttons on the seat of my trousers.

I button both buttons, satisfying his sense of order, symmetry.
I cannot button my buttons now without thinking about him.

"And the first thing we will do...."

"And the first thing we will do is bring Jay home."
So said Ann, consenting to marry me.
Her drive toward family, toward inclusion,
These and her vision impelled us.

We acted on it, bringing him home,
Including us in our family and circles,
Making him the person who enlivened our teaching and writing.

We sought control over his quality of life
By having him in our family,
Or in the loving embrace of his friends.

Ann feared having to do my role in Jay's life,
And I, hers.
I, the logistician, accountant, lawyer.
She, the gleaner of people, gathering them in, harvesting them for Jay.

We had found comfort in a division of labor,
We had feared for Jay and ourselves
When one of us would predecease the other.
But Jay died first, ending our fears.

A Failed Assumption

Ann and I recall a conversation about wonderment and Heaven:
How to tell Jay that Dad is in Heaven, if I predecease Ann.
Tell him in terms he understands: "Dad is in Heaven with Baby
    Jesus."
He would respond: "Smoking a pipe with Baby Jesus and Grand-
    daddy Turnbull."
And Ann would add, "And singing *Bye Bye Blackbird* with Grand-
    mommy Ruthie."

Then, the whole burden would be on Ann.
She has admonished me: "Don't die before I do. I can't do your job."
We assumed one would die, then the other, leaving Jay to Amy and
    Kate.
But Death undid our assumptions and freed us all to create a new life
And make new assumptions.

Primogeniture

The instinct of primogeniture has found harbor
In my DNA: To carry on "the line."

It is a family custom
To preserve the ancestral name by using it,
Not letting it lapse, die,
Re-membering the one who was
By naming the one who is.

I cannot adhere to that tradition,
Proclaim yet another Rutherford Turnbull.
There have been other sons in my life, not blood-sons, but sons
    nonetheless.
They have provided a quasi-fealty to that ancient rule.

But I have Amy and Kate, my two strong daughters
And they carry Ann's and my blood and my name.
That fact and their good lives are the sources of my joy.

Rejoicing in them and writing about Jay must be the acts
That discharge the obligation of primogeniture.

34
Letting His Light Shine
(March–April, 2009)

Unoccupied Space

With Jay, joy was more joyous.
When joy inhabited him, he would raise both arms into the air:
Jay's "Victory" sign, given with both arms, not, Churchillian, with two
    fingers.
Joy required a full-body gesture, nothing less.

On the evening of the day before Jay died, he sang his next-to-last song:
"Swing low, sweet chariot, coming for to carry me home."
Did Jay know?

Did he have a sense of the Divine?
Uncluttered by daily lives like ours, was he able to hear,
To sense more acutely the Divine?
What was he hearing when, so often,
He stared away from others, into seemingly unoccupied space?

Letting His Light Shine

On his last night of life,
Sarah, his music therapist, suggested a happier song.
They sang happily together:
"You are my sunshine, my only sunshine…
Do not take my sunshine away!"

Was he asking for his sunshine to remain,
Was he telling us to keep his sunshine?

I exchange the "u" with an "o,"
Composing a funereal version of a giddy love-song.

Kate eulogizes Jay, recalling another favorite song:
"This little light of mine, I'm going to let it shine."

I see a different light:
A chariot of fire, instantly taking Jay away,
Leaving behind his light.

35

The Evidence of Heaven and
the Power of Faith
(January–Summer, 2009)

Conjuring an Arrangement in Heaven

Ann still wants to arrange his life in Heaven.
She conjures the encircling spirits of those he knew:
Her father, my mother and father,
And of others in our lives, in our cause – especially her mother,
And commands them: be with Jay.

She wants all to be good for Jay there, as here:
Her will be done in Heaven as on Earth,
As her will for him was done here.

The Evidence of Heaven

Amy, Kate, Ann, and I have talked about Heaven.
We have asked: What is Heaven? Is it God's presence?
What does that mean?
A community of spirits?

Is it where the earthly body and person are made whole?
If so, it transforms Jay, and I ask:
Is that what he wants, what we want?

Or is it a place where there is only the present,
Just pure being, no future,
Just the eternal presence of God and loved ones,
A conjunction of spirits and joyful presence?

It is a place of light, not dark, a place of peace, not strife.
That is how Jay would have it.
That is the message his apparitions bear.

Heaven is what we wish it to be for the departed.
It is our imagination of what we want for ourselves.

The Evidence of the Divine

We have had evidence of the Divine,
Proof there is more than this world and our lives.

Ann's mother "saw" the end and spoke of it as she lay dying.
"I'm moving to another plane and it is pure love."
She has been our most reliable source, our agent of comfort.

At my father's funeral, Jay sang Dad's farewell anthems,
"The Twelve Days of Christmas,"
"Battle Hymn of Republic."

Jay gave his tinker toys, shaped like a pipe,
For Dad to take to Heaven and smoke with Baby Jesus.
 "Grand-daddy Turnbull is in Heaven,
"Smoking a pipe with Baby Jesus."
Not just a pipe, but Jay's.

There were butterflies when Amy and Kate were born,
Butterflies at the funerals for Ann's mother and father.

These symbols, these understandings,
Re-establish my faith.

The loss of loved ones brings me back to belief and faith,
Away from the edges of skepticism.

Faith quarrels with darkness.
Grief abates, becomes Mourning, but does not vanish.
Now, she is diminished, not yet vanquished, by Faith.

Bereavement, Proof of Love, and Faith

Without love, there is no pain;
Without Death, no bereavement.

The curse of love lies in Death.
Its blessing resides in the here and now
And in Faith, sorely tested and then strengthened.

Faith – that expectedness based on evidence from the past –
Is part of my response to Jay's life and death.
Faith that I will understand, if only partially,
That I will accept, if only partially,
That I will never forget, never stop re-membering.

I repeat the memorized refrains of the ancient hymns.
"Thy will be done" seems sensible, reasonable.
I find reasons why Jay died when he did.

The sense of his death, the reasons for it, explain,
And, like the artifacts and photographs, comfort,
But not enough.

Family, too, fills the open-ness, the emptiness.
A diminished family, to be sure,
But still, as always, family.

The Power of Faith

There are Providential understandings,
Intimations of the Divine,
In Jay's death.

I think about mysteries – God's –
That I cannot understand.
I accept, and I move on.

It is now – and always has been – a matter of faith.
Divinity. Providence. Grace.
Comfort, *cum forte*: strength.
These are the words that come to me.
They are words of hope and faith.

Faith sustains. She bears us on her back,
Making bearable the otherwise unbearable.

Lessons

What remains is the disembodied Jay.
That which we call his spirit.
I wish it would speak clearly to me,
Answer, "Why did Jay have to die?"

Is it because his work was done,
His life as perfect as it could have been in this world?

Was his leaving timed to tell us, as Ann has concluded,
This is the best it can be?
To teach us more lessons about how we must live?
He was our best professor, often testing before giving the course.
Has he done that again?

If so, it is not only Jay who teaches and tests,
But also God.

For Jay was God's gift to us
And God's calling Jay, "Come now, Jay, for My will shall be done,"
Must be the reason.

No other reason works.
Every other one lacks meaning:
The medical fact is just a fact,
Not an explanation.
A son's heart fails, a son dies.

Why? The answer cannot rest in biology alone.
Jay's extraordinariness was not the only gift.
It was what we and others made of it.
Death is a gift only when we can understand "why?" and "now what?"

Who, what, when, where, how? We learn the answers.
Why? That is unknown and, being unknown,
Must be answered:
Death as the will of the divine,
As Providential.

If Not for Faith

If not for Faith, then only biological reductionism.
That is not enough.
Love abides. Faith abides.
Abide with me, Ann.
Abide with us, Amy and Kate.
I ask, and each answers: I will
Abide with us, Jay.
I ask, and I know he answers: I will.

Destinies

Many times Ann and I ask,
Was Jay part of a plan?
We answer: Yes.
Was he an opportunity given to Ann, Amy, Kate, and me?
A fate-shaper?
Yes, to that, too.

He was a potential destiny that we made real, brought to life.
Biblically, we were given a choice.

Ann speaks:
"As a child, I wanted to do something in my life, to be called to
      embark on a mission,
To follow God's calling, but I had stipulations."
As a child she had not yet stipulated Jay's life, though it would become
      her mission,
Nor, as an adult, his death, a time for renewal of a new mission.

Preludes to Easter Sunday
(April 7, 2009)

Jay comes to me in a dream on Tuesday, the seventh of April, the date
    he died,
Three months ago.

He is lying in bed and will not get up. I try all my tricks. None works.
I become angry and pull his covers off.
He falls to the ground, dead.

The next day, Wednesday, I am awash in grief, and tears flow freely,
Passover begins, but I cannot pass over the past and Grief.
Past and Grief confront me, and with them are a familiar kin, Anger.

Easter and Its Promise
(April 22, 2009)

On Easter Sunday, early in the morning, light is just breaking,
I have retreated to Jay's room for sleep.

I look to the window and there, behind the gossamer blinds,
Is a shadowed cross, the frame for the windows, a presence of the
    Spirit, of Jay.

Ann and I return to Plymouth Church.
The sanctuary is full, as it was for Jay's funeral.
Only one seat is unoccupied. It is the one next to us,
The one Jay would have sat in.

Ann and I envision him, conducting the Alleluia choruses.
Our memories make him present, vital, alive, beckoning us:
"Come into joy from sadness," the hymn proclaims.
But that journey to joy is arduous.

We sing about the risen Christ, and I think:
If Christ, then, so, too, Jay:
Now I anticipate, for the first time, joining him again,
Free of my body and this life, able to be with him on his and God's
    terms.

And so I believe: Jay has risen,
But death's sting is still sharp.
Life after Death: Yes, there is evidence of it, for Jay's spirit abides in us,
Concrete, tangible in its effects on us physically and spiritually.

Till We Meet Again

We close the service as we always do,
Singing our congregational prayer:
"Smite death's spreading wave before you,
God be with you till we meet again."

I wish to smite Death but cannot.
I am conflicted:
I need to smite, but I want to remember
And fear that, in smiting, in having the triumph of my life over Jay's
    death,
I will lose Jay, lose his spirit.
And then I find the reassurance: Jay and I will meet again.

36
Living the Question
(March and April, 2009)

Intermission

How, now, shall I communicate with Jay?
I once did communicate by the little intimate gestures, made public:
Our hands-on-hip march down the hallways,
Our public repairing of un-tucked-in shirts,
And by others too, not seen by the public, hidden from others, known
    to Jay and me alone.
Now, how to have a shared being-ness with him?

This time is my interim, an intermission
Between what I had done for 41 years and what I will do hereafter,
A hiatus, a time for inwardness, introversion.

My future is occluded.
So is Ann's.
Who will be the rationale of our future together,
What will give warrant, justification to it?

The answer lies in three words: Ann, Amy, Kate.
Family is all, and always has been.

An Autumnal Purgatory

If I was increasingly care-less before Jay died,
So now I am Jay-less
And care all the more for my inward journey, my interiority.

I must find a way to find a new exteriority.
I have lost one identity and now must find a new one,
The one that Jay's death creates, the life without him.

This middle place is a purgatory for expelling what was not good
    enough,
For finding what can and should be better.

His death declares:
You, too, are in the autumn of your life.

Open to the Extreme

Ann observes:
"Jay almost never did anything to the max.
"He pushed the limits of the maximum, but never exceeded them.
"So, why the fatal, sudden, painless heart attack?
"So unlike him. Why?
"And why such swiftness in a man constantly so slow?"

To teach us to be open to the extremes?
To be ourselves, more extreme, candid in our work?
To be angry, and to be amazed by the love Jay evoked?
To acknowledge Jay's effect on the parishioner who never spoke the
Lord's Prayer
Because she wanted to hear Jay recite it?

Embracing All

We must embrace what happened, in all its complexities.
We must go down into what happened. Allow it to be in us.

To honor Jay is to take in the whole experience,
All the grief and relief,
All the joy of Jay and the horror of his death,
All the contemplation of life hereafter, of Heaven.
Mourning invites a reaching out, an embracing of the known and
　　unknown.

Grief and Mourning

Mourning is a constant presence.
Unlike Grief, she is always with me.

Grief comes and goes
She is transitory.
As much as I hate her,
I welcome her, her power to make me feel her power, to be alive
　　thusly.

But Mourning is forever at my side.
She takes my arm as I go through the motions of living,
Amused at my attempts to normalize the un-normalizable.

And just when I think she and I have accommodated to each other,
She turns me around a corner
And I meet my old friend and nemesis, Grief.

Grief's Sisters

In her company are her sisters:
Emptiness. Weariness.
Disbelief and Anger.

All feelings enlarge my emptiness.

There was a time when I thought Peace had come,
But I was wrong, and knew it.
So I accepted Resignation, a weak cousin to Peace.

But Resignation did not stay awhile. She came and fleeted away.
In her place, another old friend, Disbelief.
The cognitive dissonance: knowing but not believing.

The Silk Pall of Weariness

Weariness is a sister of Fatigue.
Like Fatigue, she saps my strength.
Elements of vitality flee.

But Weariness has a sort of lightness to her touch.
She is unlike the quilt of Fatigue, which is heavy.
She is gossamer, a silk pall.
She covers all of me, not just my body, which Fatigue attacks,
But my energy and mind, too.

Depression

Her cousin must be Depression,
That pure down-ward-ness,
Constant pressure toward the center of myself,
That compressing of all feeling toward my core.

Missing-ness

Missing-ness lies over me.
I cannot shake it off. It is too heavy.
It is unlike the sharpness of Grief and Disbelief.
Heavier than Mourning and Sorrow,
Longer-lasting than Shock and Disbelief.
It permeates; it has become part of me,
Even as Jay was my son and my best friend.

He and I had our ways,
And now his way is to make me miss him more than ever
    since he died.
When will missing-ness be lifted?

Give me some other feeling.
Bring back Shock, Disbelief, Anger, Grief, Mourning, and Sorrow.
Give me Peace and Recognition.
I petition for any feeling except the cloud of absence, of missing-ness.

These feelings, these emanations
Swirl like clouds in a storm, inconsistent, unpredictable.

Denying Jay's death denies his life.
Yet Denial reigns, a phantom warrior in the legion of missing-ness.

Pain, the Price of Love, and
Grief, the Condition of Devotion

Grief does not simply quit me.
It hides and then peeks out of its sanctuary,
And I chase it again, wanting the hurt,
For hurting means I am living and loving.

Pain is the price of Love,
Grief, the condition of devotion.

Damnation

Anger, pure vulgarity-provoking anger.
I want to say, I cannot help saying,
"God damn it."

The curse is warranted, of course,
And shameful, too.

Change the structure of the sentence,
Add a comma after "God"
And then it's a proper curse:

"God, damn it."
The "it" being Jay's merciful death.

How full of paradox is this feeling:
Damning that which is blessed.

Androgenous Anger

Anger – oh, it's there, an androgenous being.
The anger at loss – such a euphemism for death,
Such a word of false deniability for death is so real –
Has a femaleness, a gentle, almost kind, dissembling of reality,
A mask, as if applied carefully at a dressing table.

I, however, am a man, and, unlike a mother,
I did not conceive through my body,
Carry within my body,
Deliver out of my body,
Suckle and nourish through my body.

I did not lose my life-giving essences,
Those female vitalities.

But I did give care to Jay for all but three of his 41 years.

The care that was so maternal in so many ways –
The touching, the handling so he would be clean and presentable.

That was like nursing – not with one's breasts, but with one's hands.
And it was intimate, for Jay allowed me access to parts of him
That he forbade to all others.

But anger has its male side, its explosive,
Vulgarity-filled, physical knocking-about side.
It erupts: Anger that Jay is dead.

Anger at God? Perhaps, but I try not to accede to that anger.
Anger simply that Jay is not here any more.

Gone. No body to touch, no more physicality.
The ache for him becomes anger at his absence.
Anger explodes within me.

Death is the object of my anger.
If I could grab and throttle and strangle it,
If I could kill Death itself, I would

Then, Anger would bid adieu, a-Dieu.
Would say, "Until God."
But God has come and Jay has gone,
So Anger has brought me back to God.

Anger and Wonderment

Anger hides with Grief.
He is her brother.
I welcome both, in equal measure.

Wonderment is there, too.
Wonderment that Jay meant so much to others,
Was the inspiration for us and them.

And with wonderment, there is a twin, wonderfulness.
Full of wonder, of puzzlement.

"Why did Jay have to die?" Ann asks.
I have my reasons, nearly a dozen.
All rest on imperfect understandings.
But they are reasons nonetheless.

Reasons about him, about us, and, of course, about God.
Jay's life had significance
So his death must, too.

37
Physicality
(March, 2009)

Just One More Day

I cannot deny my physical heart.
The diagnosis of the last two weeks:
Heart risk, stroke risk.
Like Jay, I now have a heart problem.
Ann fears my death.

"Just one day more than my son,"
Was my measure while Jay lived:
A simple metric for how long I wanted to live.

Now, that measure becomes terrifying
As the blow that took Jay away
Lurks for me, frightening us all,
For I have had my own mild – but nonetheless real – heart attack.

The Organs of Love

With the diagnosis come two powerful medications.
The one thins the blood: watch for bleeding and bruising.
The other slows down my heart.
The medications threaten impotence.
How ironic:
One organ of love preserved,
The other jeopardized.

38
Relativity and Love
(March 24, 2009)

Ann and I married 35 years ago today.
I am blessed.
Ann, Jay, Amy, and Kate.

Four of us.
There had been five.

Five minus one is not four,
It is zero in one part of my heart,
The Jay part.

Not that I loved him more than I loved Ann, Amy, and Kate.
Or that I loved any of them more than the other.

Love is not a relative matter,
It is not susceptible to metrics.
Its quantity is immeasurable,
Its quality – the nature of the love for one person – describable.

To repair a broken heart I turn again to my family,
To Ann, and then to Amy and Kate,
And I thank God for each of them, and for Jay.

39

Returning to Native Soil, Revisited by Symbols (April 16-19, 2009)

Home-Coming, Home-Going

It is reunion time of my college class and I return
To Homewood, the name of the campus.
Homecoming to Homewood includes a renaissance
Of friendships and memories.

It is a week after Easter, the season of purple,
A time for resurrection, grief, sorrow, hope, and faith.
The timing is exquisite.

A Second Burial

Homecoming entails burial,
For a portion of Jay's ashes, contained in a small steel vial inside a
      purple velvet bag,
Have come with me, homeward bound.

Ann and I go to the family gravesites just outside of Baltimore
And gaze once again on the headstones
That memorialize three generations of Turnbull ancestors.

My father Henry and my mother Ruth are buried here,
Two parents, gathered in a single plot,
Named on a single gray stone,
Together in death, though not always, and often contentiously, in life.

A row behind them lie my grandfather and grandmother.
And behind them, my great-grandfather and great-grandmother
And their brothers, sisters, and cousins.

Today, it is Jay's turn to be reunited with his Turnbull family,
Returned to the state where he was born, this Maryland soil.

Nourishing the Family's Soil

The grave-digger fashions the hole, just a pace beyond Mother's
    remains.
It is a good hole, a foot square and a foot deep.

Ann takes the vial with Jay's ashes from me,
Holds and kisses it.
I take it from her, imagine Jay alive within it, and
I put it gently into the hole.
Both of us weep.

The grave-digger replaces the soil, scatters seed over the spot,
    and leaves.
Ann and I hold each other and our tears commingle,
Falling to the ground, nourishing the refreshed soil over our son.

Butterflies and Blackbirds

We are alone.
Or nearly so.

To the left of the Turnbull Family headstone
There is a small white butterfly.
It flitters around the cemetery,
Not landing on the headstone, but circling it and us.
Now a blackbird – a raven – alights on another headstone, closer to us
    than the butterfly.
It faces us, perched, anticipatory,
Silent and still.

Butterflies surrounded Ann's mother as she was laid down in the red
    Georgia soil.
They visited Kate on the day we brought her home after she was born.
They came to Ann's father as he joined her mother in the same soil.

Their image adorned the stained-glass ornament we saw
When Amy and Kate came home to us weeks after Jay died.

We have a photograph of Jay sitting on my mother's lap.
They are in a chair in the garden of her apartment building.
She is laughing, and Jay is reaching up to touch her face.
They have been singing.

Jay sang only one song when he spoke of mother:
"Shut the doors and light the lights,
I'll be home late tonight, bye, bye, Blackbird."

A song that created such mutual delight
And featured a bird colored as the night
Now is the song Ann and I speak together,
Holding hands and crying deeply.

Lifted on the Butterfly's Wings, Sung Away by the Blackbird's Anthem

Once again, Jay has messaged us,
Just as he did when he sang "Kumbaya"
While we debated whether to marry,

Just as he did when we buried my father,
When "Twelve Days of Christmas" and "The Battle Hymn of the
    Republic"
Were his sung tributes to my father.

We do not seek explanations of these visitations
For we know what the butterfly and blackbird mean:
Risen spirits and musical risings.

There are mysteries in Jay's life and death,
And we cannot solve them,
But only receive the solace of familiar symbols.

I have come home to Homewood, had my Homecoming,
Visited my Father and Mother and generations before them.

Jay is having his, too, his posthumous Homecoming,
Entombed with his family,
Lifted on the butterfly's wings
And sung away by the blackbird's anthem.

40

Closings of a Different Kind
(May, 2009)

An Unfamiliar Peacefulness

There is a strange, unfamiliar peacefulness this May morning of Jay's
    year of Death.
Strange because it is so calm, so pacific.
Unfamiliar because it has come to me for the first time.

The peacefulness has acceptance within it,
And a harbinger of closings.

I can walk into Jay's room and look at photographs of him as an adult
And not turn away in sorrow and anger.
That is the acceptance.
And acceptance brings a glimpse of closings.

Yet how transitory the peacefulness is.
I still find my old friends, Grief and Anger, at my side.

"There are no closings, yet," they say.
And as they speak, they precipitate my tears,
The old familiar ones, of great sorrow.

Peacefulness has its companion,
Its counter-punctual sister: Sorrow.

There is no music for Anger.
Jay and I never knew that kind of music.
And that was good, for harmony cannot come from anger,
And we had harmony.

The Past

I turn inward in my solitude,
And turn backward in time,
To these last two years.

The angry blues of 2007 and 2008,
The anxiety and the depression of the same time.

The utter physical fatigue was more than physical.
It was emotional, too:
There was no satisfying liveliness in the livelihood I had pursued.

There was a vacuum, an open-ness.
I awaited, sought the shape that would fill the void.

Filled and Enlarged

I found it: Death.
And, with it, still darker shapes on the screen.

Physical shock,
Disabling my gait, sleep, eating, thinking.
Emotional shock, blanking out other emotions,
Then receding to them.

Grief of a sort I had never known or imagined.
Yes, there was grief when Dad died, but it was brief,
Though my respect and love for him were not.

And then larger grief when Mother died,
The enlargement caused by the greater closeness we had over the
    years,
By my presence as life left her.

And sorrow when A-Dad died,
Vitality ebbing out of him as I held his hand.
As with Mother, I could feel Death and it power to rob,
And its power to fill me fully with itself, and it alone.

Pain

But with Jay: Grief such as I have never known.
Wailing, uncontrollable wailing.
No words except "I want my son back, I want Jay back."

Tears upon tears upon tears,
The exponentiality of them,
Evidence of pain,
But also producing pain.

Real physical inside-of-me pain,
The stomach-grabbing, heart-stopping pain.
I struggle to breathe.

41

Questions and Answers
(May, 2009)

Top of His Game

Throughout the winter, spring, and summer of the year of Jay's death,
Ann asks,
"Oh, Jay, why did you have to die?
"I want you to take your shower, dress, and come to work.
"Oh, Jay, I wanted to be with you when you died.
"Why did you have to die now?
"Why did you have to die when we are alive?"

We find an answer:
He left at the top of his game,
His joy quotient at its highest.

Other answers come to us, each resting in the spiritual:

To free us of worry
To prepare Ann and me for the other's death
To prepare Amy and Kate for our deaths
To be spared the long sickness he could not tolerate

To teach us a lesson about how we should live
To put us onto a different personal path
To reinforce my inwardness
To test our faith
To enliven our faith

Perhaps there are other reasons, many other ones.
Perhaps there are none we can discern,
None to which there is any sense.
Ann keeps asking, "Why did Jay have to die? And why now?"

At Least for a While

His future was secure
At least as long as Tom and Laura were able.
His job secure for at least as long as a year.
His friendships solid and many,
At least until the young people move away.
His sisters relatively settled,
At least for a while,
Ann and I in a transition mode at work,
At least for a while.

All this, at least for a while.
T'was ever thus with Jay.

Just

Just –

One more goal to set and attain,
One more objective to accomplish,
One more evaluation of our work for Jay to be had,
One more bureaucracy to be satisfied,

One more care-giver to find and train,
One more person to instruct, "Go at Jay's speed,"
One more day of doing for him, with him.
One more day of doing for ourselves, so we could do for him.

Death put an end to the corporeal Jay,
And to "At least for a while."
And to "Just one more."

Not Working for Death

Jay did not have to work to die.
Nor did we have to work in his dying.

We had worked for so much for so long,
And, now, no more.
Jay was the first of us, in death.
Jay was the fastest of us, in dying.
First and fastest were never his ways in life or in living.
In death and dying, he lead the way.
How can that be?
Death without labor, without all of the history that attended Jay,
Without "At least for a while" and "Just one more."
Why this kind of Death, which contrasts so greatly with Jay's life?

Mercy and Reward

Surely, Mercy – the swift, painless, unforeseen, unforeseeable blow of
    Death –
Is one answer to the question "why?"
There is another answer, though, one hard to speak:
Death was a reward.

A reward? Yes.

For Jay's having lived as he did, inspiringly.
For our having responded to him as we did,
Laboriously, yet gratefully.
To die the way Jay died
Is for him to be rewarded for having lived as he did,
And for us to be rewarded for our labors.

"No more work, no more worries," said our friend.
"Job well done," she said.

How to explain the sense of reward?
How to explain the preliminaries – all the readiness?
Consider:

Leaving at the top of his form.
Dying before yet another confrontation with
"At least for a while" and "Just one more".
And dying instantly, painlessly, without fore-knowledge,
Without even a present knowledge.

Grace

I cannot explain Jay's death except by attribution,
By reference to my faith,
By hearing and speaking the ancient prayer:

"The grace of our Lord Jesus Christ,
And the love of God
And the fellowship of the Holy Ghost,
Be with us all evermore."

Grace, Love, Fellowship.
Being with us all –
With Jay, and so with Ann, Amy, Kate, and me –
Evermore.

I know no other explanation,
No other sense-making of Jay's death.

I had doubted,
Even as recently as a year ago.
I had asked: Do I believe there is a God?
Now I find the answer: There must be.

And yet, in that year of asking,
In that year of contemplating my own death,
I had begun the preparations for Jay's life.
All was in readiness – for life.

Fiercely Penetrating, Vigorous Death

In its effects on us,
Sudden and unexpected death is so different than prolonged and
expected death.
It penetrates toward our souls with fierce and seemingly unrelenting
vigor,
It leaves us with so much grief that we think we can no longer bear to
live.

But of course we do live, and we go on and must go on.
Occupation with our own life blunts our pre-occupation with Jay's
death.
It is only in moments of solitude or with Ann
That I open up.
Safety permits the openness.
Solitude and semi-solitude are part of the safety, but not all of it.

Until, No More

In mid-winter through late-spring of the year of Jay's death,
I clean out my office, launching yet another edition of a book.
The activity is healthy, an antidote to the ordinariness of my work.
Until ....

Until I come across photos of Jay, Ann, and me.
He is seated between us, smiling, his face centered,
His head oversized, his very presence commanding.

I discover a letter of nearly a year ago,
Detailing the bureaucracy's inane intrusions into my and Jay's life.
Anger seizes me:
Jay is gone. No more photographs to be taken.
And no more damned meddlesome civil servants.
No more.
Oh, to have the once-again time again.

Strange words, "Until ...," with its ellipsis,
And "No more," with its thought-ending period.
The one anticipates, looks ahead.
The other closes a matter.

It will be like this for a long time,
These sequential anticipations and endings.

42

Waiting for the Future
(May and June, 2009)

The Hour Glass

A year has passed since I saw, clearly and immediately,
The end of the Center as we then knew and had created it.
As my colleagues and I struggled to secure funding for our colleagues
    and Center,
I sensed that we would not prevail:

The rooms in the hallways became empty in my mind,
Even though they were robust with people and activity.

I cannot explain this clairvoyance, nor others,
Certainly not the acts I took to prepare for the ending
That came so horribly to Jay and my family.

It is as though my life has been sand in an hour glass.
The broad half-vase seems to be the Center at its greatest strength,
Into which all the sand has been put.

Bit by bit, grants elude us, people leave us,
And the sand spills out, passing through the narrow opening,
Leaving increasingly fewer and fewer people.

They are my protogees, my students, my friends,
Headed into lives without me.
They leave me behind, not willingly but compulsorily.
There are but a few left, and soon they will depart,
Leaving the bottom vase of the hour glass nearly empty.

Re-borning

I am an old self weighted down with the past,
Lacking the old energy, purpose, and goals,
Prepped but not fully ready
To start again, yet another passage, another journey, another life.

Newborns rest, so they may grow.
So, perhaps, this old-born, re-borning self.

Open-ness and Rebirthing

Nor is it bad to have no known purpose.
Openness – the vacuum, the emptiness – is abhorrent to my nature
Yet necessary for the rebirthing.

Definite goals will come when energy returns and purpose is
rediscovered.
The renaissance will arrive.

I have circled back to a year ago,
Like sand, leaving one container, one world,
And entering another, it, too, to be left for a new world.

I have the instinct to leave work and home,
To have, if only for a few weeks, a room of my own,
Where I may allow my old self
To find a new shape, a new self.

43
Headstones and Harmony
(June and July, 2009)

No Borders

In June, I visit Jay's newly laid headstone.
His – ours – is different than all others:
Red, with no borders separating our names – Ann, Rud, and Jay.
So it was in life, so now on the red marble: no partitions, no borders.

Three names, from left to right, Ann, Rud, and Jay.
Only Jay's dates are complete: birth and death.
Mine and Ann's await our end dates.
I walk away, no grief, no sorrow, no mourning, no anger in me,
Empty.

Water
(June 24, 2009)

This is Jay's birthday, his 42nd.
He comes to me early in the morning.
I can feel him next to me in bed,

Reach to hold him, and grasp only air.
I shower in grief; there is water everywhere,
Much of it from me, not artificially poured onto me.

The Jay Tree
(June 24, 2009)

Amy and Kate take us to our university buildings.
We walk down the street; a crowd has gathered outside.
They circle around a newly planted tree.

"This is the Jay Tree," my daughters say.
It rests on the hillside between the two buildings where Jay worked.

"Let's all sing Happy Birthday," say Amy and Kate.
And we all begin to sing. I complete part of the song,
And dissolve at its end.

Jay's sisters have memorialized him,
Friends have gathered,
There is music.

It is as Jay would have it,
Precisely as he would have it.

Room for Two More
(June 24, 2009)

Later that day, we visit his grave,
Amy and Kate for the first time,
Ann and I, again.

Amy and Kate listen in silence as I say,
"The headstone has room for more names."

They know my meaning.

We contemplate our mortality, each silent.
The sun blazes, a black bird circles around us,
A small butterfly, more moth-like than others, flutters nearby.

Reconciliation, Harmony, and Congruency

I have sought reconciliation.
An apt word, at least now, at last, some four and one-half months
post-mortem.
To restore to harmony, to make consistent and congruent, to submit
to the unpleasant.

There is increasing harmony:
I begin to see the end of this meditation on Death.
Other meditations await: those about me, without the living Jay.

I discern congruency, the natural rhythm of life and death.
And I have submitted to Jay's death:
It is so absolute, so beyond my control.

I have ample mindfulness, plentiful awareness of my world and self.
It's the incongruous feelings for which I have no fondness:
I miss the man, not the duties attendant to his life.

I have written about "reward" and "relief,"
But now that the headstone is in place over him,
I sense the relief all the more.

He is laid down and covered decently,
As if he were abed in my home, and I, the laying-him-down father.

For now, for this day, I sense reconciliation.
And I welcome it.

Perhaps reconciliation is the meaning in Jay's answer, "I'm fine."
Perhaps peace and reconciliation are filigreed gold, the fine ore.
Time is telling me: it is so.
Time is healing, even as faith and love have healed.

Reconciliation flees when confrontation comes:
My voice shakes, my eyes water when I speak of Jay.
Receiving tributes to him,
I try to be calm, steady, rational, but fail.
I am no actor, no disguiser of myself.

I look at photographs of Jay as a youngster,
Laughing with Kate and Amy, dancing with his friends Suzanne and
    Sarah,
And I ask myself in disbelief,
"Was that, the photographic image,
How he truly was? Was that our life?"

Tissues and Tea
(July, 2009)

It is July in Ireland. On the western shore in Dingle,
There is a chapel famous for its stained glass windows.

I go to it, and gaze on four scenes,
Fixated upon the one of Mary Magdalene and Christ at His Tomb.
He is risen, she does not recognize Him at first.
He makes himself known to her.

Jay now makes himself known to me.
He is not visible: there is no image, no visage.
But he – his physical self – stands just outside of me,
And then enters me.

Penetrated, I am with him again.
I feel him inside me.

We are one with each other.

He makes me bear witness to my faith.
Apostolic: "the Resurrection of the body, and Life Everlasting."
Niceneic: "And I look for the Resurrection of the dead,
And the Life of the world to come."

I cannot staunch my tears.
Grief and Faith, these companions of the living who come with
     Death,
Are the married mysteries.
A guide hears my wailing and climbs the stone stairs to the chapel.
I say, "My son has died."
She offers tissues and tea.

For Jay, waffles, or cereal and milk, sufficed.
For me, on this promontory of Ireland, ripe with symbols,
Sufficiency consists of tissues and tea.

The Seventh Day of the Seventh Month (July 7, 2009)

This is an anniversary day, this July 7.
Last night, the moon was full,
And Jay danced with the angels, lighting it for us to see.

I eat where he and his friend Tom always ate,
And take away an egg roll and fortune cookie.

I go to his grave, tear away the grass that obscures the "Jay" on the
     stone,
And place the food under his name.

Tears elude me; sorrow does not, nor gratitude.
I walk to the nearby university endowment association's offices,

And make family gifts,
Some for the graveyard,
Some for a tree to be implanted into soil he trod.

There is a sense of completion in these gestures,
A harbinger of life after Jay.
Welcoming that harbinger, I also curse it,
For with Jay living, there would be no such foretelling.

"Breathe some"
(September 7, 2009)

On the precise day of the ninth month after Death came,
I take gifts to Jay,
Laying egg rolls and fortune cookies on his grave.

Two days later, workmen install the monument at the Jay Tree.

> In memory of Jay Turnbull
> KU Employee
> 21 Years.
> "BREATHE SOME."

Ann and I hold each other, oblivious to the workmen and passers by.
We weep, and, then, before we leave his tree,
We once again follow Jay:
We breathe deeply.

Out of this ceremony of death, there now comes the breath of life.

PART VI

Arcing Toward Peace

Verse is a new form for me; I am a neophyte in this style. Yet it was the form that seemed most natural, most likely to record both the facts and the emotions of the unforgettable days surrounding Jay's death.

Having written Parts IV and V, I found yet another way to write about death and more—a way that dug my interiority farther out of myself and gave it light. It was to write about myself as from afar, as though a person intimately knowledgeable about me would write. Thus, all of Part VI is in a different "person."

This "from-afar" style has been useful for expressing the arc of feelings that I found in hundreds upon hundreds of conversations with Ann, Amy, and Kate, in compassionate therapy, and in candid moments with a few old friends.

The arc began with grief, found intercession through faith, and concluded in gratitude for Jay's life and my family's love. It was an arc toward peace.

.

44

Sand, et sequitur

Sand
(August 15, 2009)

He is sand, still on the Beach,
Quiet, remaining – both kinds of stillness.

Damp, he lies there,
Waiting for the heat of a new sun,
For the life of the old son,
Perhaps for the soft breeze that will dry him,
Toss him aloft,
His grains separating, reforming, falling to a different ground.

He lifts the damp clod of himself,
Reveals some of it,
Replaces all of it,
For below that clod,
There is a netherworld,
Hinted at, barely glimpsed.

What to offer to the soft breeze,
For there is no new sun, and no son?
He awaits the answer.

The Ledger
(September 17, 2009)

Created because of a father's advice,
"Write it down, think it through,"
Because of the law's training,
"Analyze the interests, balance the equities,"
The ledger opens the man to the world,
Not all of him, not him at all times,
Just him, now.

Columns, titles italicized, like genres,
Items, like species, enumerated.

Lost:
Grants lost, Center diminished,
No larger than the day he started it with her.
Son, lost to Death,
Suddenly, shockingly, grievously.
Sense of self-worthwhile-ness, of significance,
Taken away as, in their turn, Center and Son die.

Physical assurance:
Threatened by heart troubles,
Virility depressed by drugs,
One organ saved, one nearly atrophied.

Found:
Accentuated sense of soulfulness,
Same, of mindfulness.
Similarly made more acute:
A search for completed-ness,
The acknowledgement of permanent incompleted-ness.

Welcomed:
As if from the center of the universe,

A new, more-powerful-than-ever faith,
For biological reductionism ill suits him,
And because faith makes bearable the otherwise unbearable.

Retained:
The ever-lasting, oh-so-strong sense of duty,
Obligation never to be abandoned.
Equally, the disguise that covers his true self,
That enduring pretense, that cautious with-holding.

Sought:
Something of value to fill the openness.
Much taken away, the Found and Retained are insufficient.

Advised:
Admonished to live the questions,
And to live the answers,
Therapy clothed in romanticism.
"Do that," he is advised.
"I do," he affirms.

Told:
"You are still here, not collapsed."
In agreement, he says
"I turned the bull,"
Invoking his name, his identity.

Lied:
He did not entirely turn the bull.
The charging animal – life itself –
Comes straight at him,
And he has but two choices:
Fight, and he does,
Flee, and he refuses.
The bull remains, confrontational.

Waiting
(September 30, 2009)

Live the questions, she tells him, and he does.
Live the answers, she tells him, and he does.
Or, at least those answers that come to him.
Few do.

These are not choices.
They are necessities, inevitabilities.
His life has reversed itself this year.
His son dead, his funded work vanished,
His traditional professional purposes nullified,
Or nearly so.

Directionless, he asks why
And finds reasons he does not accept:
He must still be relevant to his son's cause,
But what if he is not?

He also finds a reason he must accept:
Jay has died.

He returns to this memoir and cannot bear to read it.
He returns to the meditation and seeks to bury it.
Are those works worthwhile?
Who would care, other than him?

Tentatively, he reads and lives laterally,
Fleeing some of his present emptiness,
Probing for substance to fill the void.

He finds nothing in fleeing,
Has much in staying,
But still faces openness.

Lateralism – a sideways dodge of open-ness – does not suffice.

Action fails him.
Nor does simply being in this time and place suffice.
Inaction also fails him.

He awaits, anxious for answers.
It is not a choice.
It is his obligation.

Acute
(October 2, 2009)

The sameness of life, especially its emptiness,
Is familiar, like a friend.

He had grown accustomed to her, this lady emptiness.
Tolerance did not mean fondness, much less love.
He would have traded her, this emptiness, for vitality.

Then Death came,
And suddenly life became acute:
Emptiness vaster, a void;
All senses,
All feelings,
All understandings
Cut far more deeply into him.

Immediately, poignancy entered and stayed, like an un-sutured cut.
But in time she too bade farewell.
He knew she would leave,
And that in her place the sameness would return.

Blood coagulates on its own
And what has been is once again.

He does not wish for Death,
But for his son,

And if not for him, for that is impossible,
Then, at least, for the reason to proclaim,
"Life is acute."

There was life in the Death that cut so deeply.

Gestation
(October 7, 2009, the ninth month after January 7, the day Jay died)

Compulsorily, for his publisher,
He scans hundreds of photographs
Of his dead son.

There, memorialized for today, are the yesterdays,
And his son's sweetness and twinkling eyes.

Remembrance brings joy, delight, liveliness,
And tears, for in the nine months past his son's death,
Life has dimmed and gone flat.

Gestation of life requires nine months.
How many months does the gestation of solace require?

Nearly
(November 10, 2009)

He takes his constitutional and remembers
Not the calamity of his son's death,
But his responses.

Aware of the convolution of emotions,
Of his psychic history,
He feels none of them now.

Even disbelief – the last to leave him – has vanished.

He has begun new work, lawyer work.
A freshness seems to be entering him:
The walk in the gentle fall afternoon
And the labor to create new law
Renew him.

Until early the next morning,
Jay appears, in a dream,
Eating, happy, nearly explosive.

The dreamer reaches to touch his son,
To calm him.
The reach fails.
His son disappears,
Nearly recaptured.

Nearly empty of the earlier feelings,
Nearly starting to fill his open-ness,
Nearly touching his son,
He accedes to Nearly-ness.

It gives more solace than Far-ness,
That sense of his son's distance and absence,
That knowledge of emptiness.

Nearly-ness approximates future,
And nearly suffices.
He knows he must wait,
He is nearly what he will become.

Belief, Suspended
(Dec. 7, 2009, eleven months after Jay died)

He views photographs, hundreds of them, of his son.
Was this the baby, the boy, the youth, the man,
He asks – this, my son –
He of the blond curls and sweet smile,
He of the enlarged head,
He of the beloved and loving family?

He believes, with fullness, all these photographs tell him,
Remembers the moments they were made,
The facts of them.
He has memories of memories.
But, yet, he cannot truly believe these images, their significance.

"This could not have been my life," he thinks.
"I do not remember it, I did not experience it.
"That is some other father, some other son, some other family.
"It is not – cannot be – mine."

These preservations
Are as unreal as the days of his son's death were surreal.
He has been: the proof is in the images.
But neither has he been that man, that father.

He remembers well and can affirm the being-ness
Of all of his other histories,
But not of this one.

One part of his mind declares,
"It never happened."
It speaks for him:
"I never had the joy of Jay,
"Nor the pain."

It is as though he and Jay
Never were.

What is this strange blockade,
This repression,
This incapacity to affirm the absolute reality
Of his and his son's life?

It is not the peace, the resignation he has felt before.
This is a new friend, Belief of Personal History, Suspended.

At Ease
(January 7, 2010)

You are at ease, his friend tells him.
That is her sense of him, this anniversary day.

There is a rightness in her judgment:
He does rest more easily now.
Having confronted all those reactions to his son's death,
He has faced his life without his son and summed it:

All this is about growing old –
All the talk of remains, open-ness, carelessness about his work,
Of the quest for vitality and virility.

Yes, she agrees, but she cautions:
It is not necessary to frame yourself within a single border,
There is value in recognizing that which is thematic,
But greater value in not compounding and collapsing all into one.
Your ease is not a lack of emotions,
But a quality of comfort with them all.

He complains: I can remember my father, who left me at seven,
My mother, who raised me,

My wife and daughters, who enlivened me,
But not my son, so vividly and with such single memories
As them.

Each person except his son is sharply remembered in sequence:
From the most distant in my life to the most present.

That is the way memory works, she tells him:
The closer the person, the more the associations,
The less discrete the memory.

An explanation of his ease?
Or an explanation to ease him?
Is ease a disease?
Or is it the evidence of healing?

Anniversary
(January 7, 2010)

Confined to his home by deep snow and howling winds,
He abandons ceremonies long planned:
The conversation with his pastor, revising his discourse with God;
His talks with his friend, depleting and then refreshing himself
In the room safe for his emotions;
The visit to his son's grave and the leaving behind of candy and
    egg rolls,
The oft-enjoyed edibles of a man no longer eating,
These tributes to memory.

It has been a year now, almost to the minute,
Since Death broke in and the argument began:
The argument with God about why, why now, and how.
And the feelings, those he knew he would have,
And the ones he could not anticipate.

He vainly seeks to recapture the feelings this winter morning,

But they elude him, all but one:
The pure utter inescapable gone-ness of his son.
The emptiness, vacuum, void, openness remain.
Writing these words prompts a tear, a tremble in the face.
He has summoned the residue of a year,
Provoked feeble souvenirs of those twelve months.

He tries to remember life with Jay –
Not the events but the liveliness of their life:
The incorporeal sounds and scents, the music and dance of their days
    together.
They evade him.
He can touch his son's possessions, hear his recorded voice,
Summon through those media what has been.
These are poor surrogates for the memory that time has diminished.
All else is gone.

He kisses his wife awake,
Tells her, "There were moments."
They lie in each other's embrace,
Silent except to acknowledge together their pain,
Unspoken, but their eyes are tearful.
They do not need words.
They had him, they have each other.
That suffices for this tender moment.

That and the calls from his daughters,
The mutual restraint on tears,
The semi-forced remembrance of joy and Jay,
The affirmation that all of us ate waffles this morning,
And then, as always, the knowledge
That four of them collectively are far less than five minus one.

Haunted
(January 13, 2010)

He seeks his son's body, the scent, laughter, voice, and flapping
    fingers,
Desires to relive the days of his son's life.
His body seeks the other's,
His soul searches for the other's.
He is haunted by a quest for the corporeal
And only partially satiated by the finding of the soulful incorporeal.

Engagement
(January 15, 2010)

He dreams:
A man, in blue blazer, white shirt and red tie, sorts corn flakes.
The man is engaged, his behavior repetitive and predictable.
Is he the man?
Is his son the man?
What difference lies between them?

Engaged, his son was like him.
Engaged, he was like his son.
He remains engaged, for there is no other option.
His son's cremains lie still,
Engaging him, the remaining man.

Waves
(January 17, 2010)

In Hanalei,
The waves play
The same music every day.

He stands ashore, listening:
Where is his son's voice?

It is silent, not realized.

He tries to remember his son's voice, face, touch,
The events of their inseparable life,
And fails, hearing only the building of the waters' crest and its crash.

But he sees
White veins within the towering blue foam.

His memory gathers, builds, compounds, like the waves themselves.
It rises and then atomizes on the sandy shore of his life.

There is no single memory, no single wave independent of all others,
Just veins of memory inside the waters of his life,
Forming, compounding impartably, and then dissolving.

Decade within a Day
(January 18, 2010)

His wife has told him, sympathetically and fearfully:
You aged a decade within a day.

And so he did, that January 7, 2009.
Shocked by his son's death,
Stooped his back, halting his gait, haggard his visage.

Dead at 41,
Aged to 81 in a day:
The son and the man.

Outside of them, in her own misery,
His wife faces her son's death, sees his yellow body, kisses his cold lips,

And witnesses her husband age a decade within a day.

Gone is the fear she had for her son's life and last days,
Replaced by the fear for her husband's
And perhaps her own.

No End
(January 21, 2010)

My son died.
I looked inside myself and found remains.
I looked outside myself and found a void.
I buried his cremains
And carried on.

Delete
(April 7, 2010)

Fifteen months have passed, to this day.

He opens his cell phone, scrolls to "J" and finds the entry "Jay."
At his office, he looks at the speed dial on his desk telephone.
There, too, is "Jay."

He knows there is no telephone service,
There will be no response.
Tom and Laura have left,
So, too, Jay, but in a different, graver way.

The blossoms on the Jay Tree have not yet come out
But the tree has greened, is pregnant with white flowers.
At Jay's home, the tendrils of the forsythia dance like ballerinas,
Daffodils smile at the heavens,
And life abounds, for the soft spring has followed the hard winter.

Is it time to finish the final deletion,
To excise the "Jay" marks on his telephone?
He wants to do it, knows he should,
But cannot.

One last reminder of the daily connection,
The speed-dials on his telephones,
Must persist.
No season-changing occurs.

These symbols are forever.

Abandoned
(April 11, 2010)

His son dies.

Everything changes.
Nothing changes.

He had written those two penultimate and ultimate lines in reverse
    order.
He had expected, eagerly pursued, studied for, even planned for a
    change.
But of what? For whom? How? Why?

Those were the questions he asked and sought to answer.
He wrote as never before: about his son, his family, himself.
Words came easily; most remained, edited;
Some, banished by their author, were unfit to live.
Words were easy to attain.
Action was elusive.

He took time from the pre-death routine to write,
To talk to himself, seen by him, the writer, from afar.

He read about other theologies, other ways of life.

But the "what" of change eluded him.
The "for whom" remained.

The "how" never came to him,
Except to quit his profession, expend his hard-gotten resources
And encounter emptiness.
His need for security forbade the "how."

The "why" he knew well:
He had done all he had expected, and more:
There truly was nothing left, no goal, no ambition,
Except to write,
To enjoy that solo mental and emotional gratification:
    Scribo, ergo sum.

Everything changes: His son is dead.
Nothing changes: He persists in his old ways.
The future is as the past.
Regret visits him as he abandons change.

Fallow
(May 12, 2010)

He is a field become fallow,
Failing in fecundity.

It is not his body that awaits fertilization
And photosynthesis.
He feeds and weeds it
And finds other nourishment apt for its needs.

The fallow-ness is in his spirit.
Ambivalent about present and prospective work,

No longer care-less – that degree of abandonment is inapposite now.
But ambivalent, capable of holding conflicting thoughts and desires,
Unsure – not of himself, not of his capacities,
But of his role.
For the first time, he is not self-reliant, not self-determining,
Rather much a stranger to himself.

"Hey, there," he greets his fallow spirit,
And receives no answer.
The silence is expected:
Fallow land is quiet, awaiting.

Egg Rolls
(July 6, 2010)

He visits his son's grave,
This day, one short of 18 months to the day after Death came,
And places on the red stone, below his son's deeply cut name and
    dates,
Two egg rolls.

"Here, Jay," he whispers,
"Are my symbols of remembrance,
One for the struggle of your life and death,
And one for the joys of your life."

He has been consumed with Death's sisters:
Grief, Sorrow, Anger, Despair, and more,
And seen the Alphas that might arise from the Omega of a life ended,
But not embraced them.

Departing from his son, he vows:
"The next symbols will celebrate your life and the joy you brought."

He pauses, corrects himself, changes the plural to singular:

No longer two egg rolls, each competing for his mind and heart,
But a full meal, brought to his son, Jay, the joy-giver.

Alpha commences today.

TIA
(July 7, 2010, anniversary of his son's death
18 months before)

He had anticipated deliberate and accidental changes in his life,
Phasing out of his work, then retiring, free to seek and find
Modest hedonism in places near and afar, in books, friends, and
    family,
And in accidental changes and surprising epiphanies, those that are
    fate's contributions.

He had not reminisced about his mild heart attack a year ago,
The threat to his heart, with family in Nashville.
Such an accident was far from his mind, for he is healthy now,
In both body and spirit.

He takes his luggage to the door of his home,
Leaving it for transport to Washington,
Bends down, deposits his bags to the floor,
And cannot stand up steadily.

He secures a purchase on the table near him,
Instinctively staggers to the kitchen, not knowing why, seeing double
    vision,
When, accident upon accident, his wife arrives.

His words slurred, he says, "Hospital … cannot walk … "
And falls, breaking his parents' antique mahogany drum table.

Ann guides him to their car, delivers him to emergency care,

Stays by him all night, as, gradually, his competencies return and he is
     released.

Alpha begins with a mini-stroke, the most unanticipated of insults.

And thus does accident trigger deliberation:
"What does this mean for the rest of his life,
"Just how long and joyful will it be?"

Joy
(July 11, 2010)

This is an inadequate word, this word "Joy."
Juxtapose "Jay" with "Joy" and the insufficiency is clear.

With Jay, there was more than delight,
More than felicity,
More than gaiety.

These triplets were often present,
Absent only during the horrid outbursts,
Abiding the long-lasting depressions.

Together, they cannot begin to tell Jay's story:
The utter, absolute up-ness, the high-ness of his son's moments with him.

There were cares, concerns for his son,
Sometimes silent,
Sometimes public,
Agents of the creation of a community of care surrounding his son,
All shared with his wife.

But no cares ever diminished the love,
Ever blunted the father's joy, his inexpressible gratitude for the gift of
     his son's life.

Joy admits an irrepressible but infrequent gasp of sorrow,
But it now surmounts Death and her sisters.

Joy trickles into the old openness,
Washes away the Omega of his son's death,
Forms the Alpha of this post-mortem life.

Joy is ultimate remembrance,
The categorical imperative of the father's future.

As If
(August 20, 2010)

They return to a Carolina island
To which they retreated after marrying.

Thirty-six years have passed,
A son has been brought home,
Two daughters birthed and raised,
And, horrifically, a son taken by death.

Standing in the Atlantic,
He looks to the horizon,
Trying to remember.

Water and sand merge as waves come ashore,
Indistinguishable, lapping at him and his memory,
Where there is no single recollection of his son.

It is as if his son had not been,
As if there had been no energy defining father and son together,
As if their co-existence were non-existence.

WWJW
(August 7, 2010)

He has tried to recapture the pain
That came
With death,
But failed.

There was a time when pain was all,
And when it was nearly all,
And now, when it is not even a gossamer pall.
If that is healing, he has wanted no part of it.

Standing in the ocean, the sun setting, the beach empty,
He concedes to painlessness
And finds a replacement in the form of a question:

"What would Jay want?" he wonders,
And finds the answer, so obvious he could not discern it until now:

Jay would want laughter, music, friends, and satisfaction with each
    day's work,
All in such surfeit that his arms would reach to the heavens,
Glorifying this life.

That is what he must have,
That is his way to honor his son:
There must be a new quality to his life,
One of joy.

That is what Jay would want.

Iron and Glass
(October 3, 2010)

It has been five years since they installed iron and glass into their home.
Three chandeliers – their three children – illuminate their hours
    together,
Alternately fully lighted, dimmed, and extinguished.

In these years, she grows into the woman she was meant to be:
As bright and colorful as the glass itself,
As firm as the iron that binds them together,
A work of art herself – a spirit and mind fused into singular beauty.

At an art auction, she fixes her mind onto an addition to their home,
A trio of primary red and blue glass globes congealed by a single
    swirling iron rod.

He, the skeptic, hesitates and then feels the familiar desire,
That internal necessity for her to be and become –
Now, to have this complement to the three chandeliers.
Acquiring them grows her loveliness even more
And brings yet more of her into his life.

He has needed her glass and iron self.
As she becomes more beauteous in these years,
He, having feasted on her, finds himself famished for yet more of her.

423
(October 28, 2010)

He spends an agonizing night.
Distraught by one therapy,
Pained by another,
Poisoned by fish,
He awakes after three hours' sleep,

Remains conscious for yet another three,
Save but for moments in dreamland.

There, he views photographs of his son,
Races to a room where his son dances alone,
Reaches toward him,
Embraces a torso,
Gives and receives a kiss,
And encounters loneliness, his son suddenly vanished.

He awakens in tears,
His breathing rapid,
His heart fibrillatory.

It is 4:23 a.m.

Celebration
(December 12, 2010)

He culls through photographs of his family,
Seeking those just right for his memoir of his son.

He celebrates the lives they record,
The memories they evoke.

And then he finds those recording
The Memorial Service,
And is met by memories and mourning.

Tears shrouding his eyes,
He holds his wife, his son's mother,
And celebrates with her the life that was and is no more.

Tendrils
(Sept 28, 2010)

Grief is stealthy.
Like a perennial in winter, she hides beneath the surface of his
    memory
Until, unexpectedly, she energizes herself, and
Locks him with her tendrils.
He escapes by watering her with his tears.

The Bird and the Brook
(January 2, 2011)

If we have ever been thrilled by the sight of a Blue Jay,
Or the sound of a laughing brook,
We can hold the thrill forever
And we will seek it always.

So it is with his son and grief:
He has been almost two years away from him,
Reconciled to the never-again-ness of life with his son,
Relieved that Grief's sensuous grip is gone,
Glad of the healing that seems to have come at last,

And now glad that the deep feeling of being-ness
Caused by Grief revisits him.

Being open to being opened
Allows him to submit to the colors and sounds
Of the man who, two years ago, he delighted to have,
And to the imprisoning power of Grief.

Being alive entails welcoming Grief
Even as it entails Delight
In his remembered sights and sounds of his son.

Masks
(May 23, Venice, Italy)

In Venice, not all is as it seems.
Masks, the theatrical disguises, abound,
Asking, when in our home as now:
What is the reality –
The sorrow or the healing,
Or, as masks are donned and shed easily,
Both?

Anniversary – 2
(January 7, 2011)

Two full years have passed, to this day.
Father and mother breakfast where their son loved to eat
And on the food that was his last word:
"Waffles."

It was always waffles,
As soft as their son's soul,
As sweet as his laugh.

They order the same,
Preserve a corner of each meal,
And visit his grave.

Against the sharp wind on this clearest of days,
They place the remains of their meal on his cremains,
Hold each other, bound in memories and gratitude,
And give thanks for his glorious life and merciful death.

Today, Grief is a stranger,
Gratitude, the intimate one,
Faith, the sustainer,
And Love, the victor.

Eulogy by Kate Turnbull

My brother used to say to himself in times of stress, or not, "Deep breath, JT. You've gotta breathe some." So, for my sake, and in honor of Jay, let's all breath together, shall we? In true Jay Turnbull fashion, I will count it off: a one, a two, a one two three...

(Breathe)
Thank you.

On behalf of my parents and my sister, I want to thank you all for being here with us. I want to thank those friends and family who have traveled from far and wide to honor my brother, those old house-mates, job coaches, Beach Center employees, and all of you who are here today. I know I can speak for my entire family when I say that the outpouring of love over the last couple of days has been, like JT himself, truly extraordinary. We also must thank Tom and Laura and the entire Riffel family for the love and care that you have given Jay for the last seven plus years. He was indeed a member of your family too.

The last time I saw Jay was over Thanksgiving break. He and I drove out to Wendy Parent's house to visit the animals. Wendy offered him a choice of four different pies and Jay had a slice of three of them. He cleaned up after himself. He pet the cats. He gave Wendy a soft-five and we were off. But the party, I'm sorry to say, Wendy, really started when we got in the car. I was blasting the soundtrack to "Hair," which was always one of Jay's favorites, and we were singing—shouting more like it. He was doing his bounce and flapping his fingers and his eyes were crossing a little like they did when he was really having a good time. But I looked over at one point (it's hard to keep your eyes on the road when you are jamming out with Jay Turnbull) and he looked at me right in the eyes and he had this little smile of joy, of contentment, of love. And I thought, "There is God. There *is* God. *There* is God."

Jay had a rather special relationship with the divine. I always imagined that angels talked to him throughout the day. You have all seen him, sitting quietly in his chair and he would suddenly, and without any outside prompting, giggle. "What's so funny, Jay Turnbull?" "Smiling," he would say. Who was he talking to? And what plans were they shaping up together for the rest of us?

He talked to God every night. These prayer sessions would vary in length and many of you were often included along with a few other special mentions. "God bless Mom and Dad. God bless Tom and Laura. God bless Aunt T and Uncle Will. God bless pancakes. God bless Grandma Dot and Mr. Jim. God bless Muncher's Bakery. God bless Brandon and Sarah. God bless cereal. And milk."

Cereal and milk. This is what mattered to him.

Getting a piece of chocolate from Michelle Longhurst after she lovingly trimmed behind his ears and washed his hair.

Pouring a package of M&Ms into a bowl and eating them one at a time. Mom and Dad would joke that that must be what paradise sounded like to him. And please, indulge me, for Jay. (pour M&Ms)

Paradise sounds like a package of M&Ms being poured into a bowl.

Paradise is a soft five.

Paradise is a place for everything and everything in its place.

Paradise is a chicken sandwich and a Sprite.

How much we mortals have to learn from the likes of Jay Turnbull.

My parents always said he was their greatest teacher but they just wished that sometimes he had given them the course before the final exam.

He was embraced by the Lawrence community in ways I know my parents did not dream possible when they first moved here in 1980. (Chip was saying that it seems so eerily perfect that they landed here, of all places. Jay's middle name was Lawrence. Our university mascot is the Jayhawk.)

But how could we not embrace him? How could we not strive to reach our highest potential as human beings when he was around? He was the best of the best. He knew no judgment, no race, no class, no sexual orientation. None of the things that we mortals see in one another, that we size up about each other.

He had no concept of shame. He would pick that nose if it needed picking, he would roll over to one side if feeling a little gassy, and when we were in a crowd of people, he would always remind me of that time-tested rule, in his very, very loud voice: "Never touch your penis in public."

How did he not see the stares around him? How did he just not care? I certainly did, especially as a child and young adult when embarrassment was the currency we all traded in.

I remember the phase when Jay Turnbull started, as my parents called it, getting a life. When he attended fraternity parties at the SAE house where, of course, a little picking and rolling would go completely unnoticed. When he moved into his own home. (It was never, ever, a house! It was always a home! How could somebody who didn't even know how to read understand that distinction?!) When Alex at Free State came to his rescue when some drunk guy was giving him a hard time in the restroom. "Don't you know who this is?" Alex said. "This is Jay Turnbull."

He never really belonged to us. He was here on borrowed time. He was an angel walking the streets of Lawrence, Kansas.

And what in the world do we do now that he is gone?

He had many songs in his life, my brother did. But one that was always a favorite was "This Little Light of Mine." "This little of mine, I'm going to let it shine. Let it shine, let it shine, let it shine."

His light shone on you. His light changed you. Indeed, after the incredible outpouring to my family these last couple of days and seeing you all here today, I cannot help but wonder if he was in fact closer to the divine than we all thought. Let it shine, those angels whispered in his ear. Let it shine.

321

And, today, this song means something even more to me. Since Jay truly knew no judgment, since he truly saw the brightest and most glorious lights in all of us, what will it take for us to live up to his example? To love ourselves with his encompassing love? To walk through life as he did, blissfully unafraid of death? To give a soft-five of friendship to everyone we meet? This is the final exam. Are we willing to be the people that Jay Turnbull had the faith that we were? Are we willing to let our light shine?

I was not done having Jay in my life. I can see him now as I did so many times over the years as I dropped him off at Haworth Hall or his home, walking away from the car, the slowest walk in the history of mankind with his feet splayed out to the sides, his shirt tucked in and, possibly, the bright, white rim of his underwear out for all to see (for what in the world did he care?).

He would walk away from me and, without ever looking back, he would raise a hand in the air and do a backwards wave. As if to say, "I've got it from here." I would often drive away at that point, knowing that as a man, and not a boy, JT didn't like his little sister watching over him. But sometimes I would watch him and just sit in gratitude, profound gratitude for the blessing he was in my life.

He never really belonged to us. And how lucky we were to have him.

He would close his marathon prayer sessions each night by saying "God bless all the good people."

God bless you, Jay Turnbull, for showing us the way. For gracing us with your presence. For shedding your light on us.

We will continue to work to be worthy of it.

Eulogy by Peter Luckey, D.Min.
Pastor, Plymouth Congregational Church
Lawrence, Kansas

The Prophet Job said,
> *The Lord giveth*
> *The Lord taketh away*
> *Blessed be the name of the Lord.*

In the life, death and life beyond death of Jay-T Turnbull, can we say blessed be the name of the Lord?

We gather as family, as community, as friends and loved ones, to grieve, to mourn, to shed tears, but finally we come to offer our deepest gratitude and love to God that God should have seen fit to bless our lives with an uncommon human being in Jay-T Turnbull.

Yes, one more time we had wanted to give and receive his secret handshake, once more wanted him to belt out a joyful "Alleluia!"

Many of us are still in a state of shock. We still have not had time to take it all in, to process what has happened … that here was JT getting ready for work on Wednesday morning, ready to dress and go off to work at the Beach Center. It is all so sudden.

So we fumble for words that are partial, incomplete, hardly able to capture a life—who JT was for us, and far beyond the scope of Lawrence, Kansas; unable to fully comprehend that, through Ann and Rud's work, lives were helped, hope was rendered, all by JT's example of what a life of one with intellectual disabilities and autism could be.

What we have known and learned through JT is the uncanny way in which those who have been short changed with tools to cope in this world seem to be endowed with a capacity to be a window to that other world.

I believe this: There are angels who walk among us and we do not know it.

It was as if, in being with him, there were always glimpses being revealed of something greater and deeper, of a love and a spirit beyond us. Let me give you an example.

Ann's mother was dying. The family is gathered around her bed at the hospital. She wanted everyone to hold hands and sing "Kumbaya." Everyone sang through the night and in the morning Ann's mother died.

Now fast forward six months. Ann and Rud met. Rud, being the wise person he is, asked her to marry him. But Ann was afraid, overwhelmed. Both had been down the marriage path before. She said, "I wish my mother were here to help me with this decision." From the other room, as Kate tells it, "My brother, my sweet, sweet brother, who had few verbal skills at this point, started to sing 'Kumbaya.' My Grandmother was there. Ann and Rud were married. The rest is history."

This was the gift of the person who walked among us.

JT was born on June 24, 1967 in Baltimore, MD. He lived in Lawrence since moving here with his family from Chapel Hill in 1980. Jay had multiple disabilities, but he was the inspiration for his parents, Rud and Ann. He motivated them to create the Beach Center, and then their teaching and their writing, learning, insight, and understanding spread all over the world.

But it was JT really… their love for him, the love they received from him… that was the source of their prodigious output.

JT was a reminder to us all that our passions and callings almost invariably have a human face, a personal experience that animates our life mission, our life's work.

It was JT who, Ann and Rud freely admit, kept them grounded.

But it was not just Ann and Rud. JT kept his sisters, Amy and Kate, the whole family, grounded as well.

When Kate Turnbull was confirmed at Plymouth some 16 years ago, she shared her faith with the congregation here in the sanctuary. And she gave credit to her brother,

Jay has taught me about God in the simplest and only way he knew how. At dinner one night, I asked him, "Jay, do you love God?"

His answer was "yes."

"Jay, does God love you?"

His answer, "Yes."

He does not question and demand an answer as to "How do we know God is here? What happens after we die?" or "Will God forgive me for doing something wrong?"

Jay is not bothered by the details of God.

He simply knows that he loves God and God loves him…. He blesses everyone he knows…. At the conclusion of his prayers he says, "And God bless all of the good people." Jay reminds me every day not to question and demand so much of God, but just to love and have faith in the Holy Spirit.

What a tribute to faith. How powerfully JT has shaped the lives of those around him and will continue to do so.

I want to close by saying a word about his Dad. Rud and Jay T as father and son were close, very close.

Like any father, Rud had the greatest of hopes for his first born son. And Rud, having been schooled in the high achievement world of New England prep schools and elite universities, knew something of the unspoken expectations for achievement, excellence, and brilliance in that fiercely competitive world.

Like many in the achieving world, Rud began his career in the legal profession. But God has a way of wrecking havoc with our vocational plans.

What does a father do with his dreams and ambitions when his son, his only son, is, by accident of birth, never going to be Phi Beta Kappa or climb to the top of the academic ladder? How does a father reorient his goals and dreams, not only for his son, but for himself?

Rud, you did both: You gave your all to JT. You gave him the best quality of life a father could ever give a son.

And as much as you shaped JT's life, JT shaped your own. Out of your deep love and empathy for him, you poured all your talents and energies into being an advocate and teacher for the world on behalf of people with intellectual disabilities. You and Ann together started the

Beach Center. He was your vocation; you were Father in every sense of the word, in the Biblical sense of the world. In the end what matters is not degrees, and achievements, but love and compassion.

You know the Father I am speaking of… the one in the story of the prodigal son. He, too, had to wrestle with dashed hopes and crushed dreams.

And yet, when it mattered, when that prodigal son came home, dashed hopes and crushed dreams did not matter. It was a homecoming of robes and rings, fatted calves, and parties because this is your son who was dead, but now is alive, was lost but now is found.

Rud, you wrote some words that I have kept for the past 13 years. It was a book review about a book called *Uncommon Fathers*. In it you wrote,

Who does not yearn for his son, his first born, and in my case only son, to carry on a legacy that at least in my family has been consistent across male generations? What father does not struggle with letting go of the ghost of the son he expected but did not have? What father, looking at his unexpected son, does not see him to be a perfect representation of his forefather?

I could feel the struggle in Rud's writing. But he ends the review with these words,

Our children are our darkness and light and in the end they are our butterflies, emblematic of our own spirits, often crushed but never dead. They will hover around our lives and our graves, incandescent, generative, and generational, ultimately reassuring.

How well you said it, Rud. Jay is the one who now hovers around our lives now… the butterfly, incandescent, as you say.

He is the light, the window into the beyond, the manifestation of God's love here among us. He was that, and is that now even still.

Angels walk among us and we never know it.

Alleluia, indeed. Alleluia!

I say Thanks be to God for the life of Jay Turnbull.

Eulogy by Michael Wehmeyer, Ph.D.
Professor, University of Kansas

Ann and Rud often said that Jay was their best professor, but that he was hard because he often gave them the final examination before giving them the class. But Jay's tutelage went far beyond that of his parents and his family. His friends and colleagues and, indeed, people from across the country and the world learned from Jay. As word spread this past week of Jay's passing, many of us in the Beach Center began to hear from people far and wide whose life had been touched by Jay. These were people who knew Jay personally, but also people who knew Jay only from the stories and pictures that Ann and Rud shared with audiences about his life.

I am reminded of the book *Power of the Powerless* by Christopher de Vinck, in which he tells the story of his brother, Oliver, who was born with severe, multiple disabilities. Writing several years after Oliver's death, de Vinck described Oliver as "the weakest, most helpless human being I ever met, but, also one of the most powerful human beings I ever met. He could do absolutely nothing," de Vinck wrote, "except breathe, sleep, and eat, and yet he was responsible for action, love, courage, and insight."

You glimpse Jay's power by the number and types of people gathered in this sanctuary and by the e-mails and letters and blogs and phone calls from around the country and around the world; in these, you sense the power in Jay's capacity to inspire others to action, to love, to take stances of moral courage, and, to gain new insights and visions for what might be possible.

The lessons Jay imparted were simple, but important in the context of our too often hectic lives. He reminded us to remember the holidays; to revel in family and loved ones; to live life with gusto; and to have favorite foods that excite you. But Jay's ultimate lesson to me came this week. When the press release announcing Jay's death was posted Wednesday night, I paused after I read the link from the KU home page to the news release. That link read: University Mourns Longtime Employee Jay Turnbull.

Think about that for a moment. The headline could just as easily have read "University Mourns Son of Distinguished Professors" or "University Mourns Special Worker." Instead the headline points out a simple fact; that Jay was a person in and of himself, independent of who his parents were or whether he had a disability. He was a person who worked for 20 years and who contributed to the mission of the Beach Center, the Life Span Institute, the School of Education, and the university.

And in reflecting on that headline, and thinking about Jay and his impact on my life and the lives of others, I realized that the most important lesson Jay taught me was not really about the possible lives people with severe disabilities can lead, that people with severe disabilities could live in their own homes or perform meaningful work or lead a full social life. Those are important lessons, I know, but these lessons are really about the business of education or the rehabilitation business or the business of the myriad of professions that provided the supports that sustained Jay.

No, what Jay taught me, and what I believe he taught so many around the world who join us today to mourn his passing and celebrate his life, was that we are not in the education business or the rehabilitation business, or any other business; we are, each of us, in the dignity business. By the quality of his character and the example of his life, Jay reminds us of the dignity of living full lives; lives rich with friends and family and the dignity of work and the security of home and the joy and gift that is each day. Tennessee Williams wrote that "Life is an unanswered question but let us still believe in the dignity and importance of the question." Because of Jay, I know more about the dignity and importance of every person. I can think of few more important lessons to have imparted or a more important legacy to have left.

Eulogy by Mary Morningstar, Ph.D.
Professor, University of Kansas

Throughout the arc of Jay's life and along the short sweep of his time with us, he touched our hearts in personal ways. In terms of how his life intersected and in many cases impacted societal views of disability, Jay was a personal emissary of full community inclusion for individuals with disabilities.

I had the pleasure of first meeting Jay and his family, Ann and Rud, Amy and Kate at his temporary home in Bethesda, MD while Ann and Rud were on sabbatical from KU. I was meeting with him and his family because for a very brief period of time, Jay was my student.

When I met with him and his family, it was a warm summer night as we sat out on their deck right before the beginning of the school year. Because Jay had just turned 20, it was to be his final year in high school. We met to discuss priorities for Jay's school program, what the family's plans were for life after high school, and what skills we were to work on for that upcoming year. I might mention that the Turnbulls hosted us with some "entertainment" for the evening.

Now I don't remember if this was planned or spontaneous, but I do remember Kate and Amy singing and dancing (Amy, I believe you were the dancer; and Katie, a budding Broadway musical star). In reflecting on that meeting, it was my first inkling of Jay's love of music and that the joy of music was not only integral to who he was as an individual, but it reflected his love for his family. And as most of you know, strains of music, laughter, and lively people have resonated throughout his life.

That year I collected plenty of data related to how Jay progressed in terms of his skills needed to prepare him for his future (I believe he achieved 90 percent accuracy using a picture recipe to microwave macaroni and cheese). However, another critical goal for Jay was to achieve the skill of "being cool and hanging out." Because I was teaching in an innovative grant-funded program through the University of Maryland which was designed to move students with significant disabilities from segregated special schools into the mainstream of regular high schools, Jay needed a few tips on how to carry his backpack (slung over one shoulder) and how to saunter down the hall. So he and one of the high school boys, who helped out as a student aide in my classroom, would "practice" walking cool and hanging out in the quad. This turned out to be a highly desirable activity for all involved, because as many of you know, Jay has always been surrounded by beautiful women, and therefore, it was a win-win situation—for Jay and the guys who supported him.

What became apparent during this year was how Jay influenced me as a teacher and as an individual. I entered teacher education right at the cusp of major changes in the field of special education; PL 94-142 (special education legislation that for the first time mandated public education for students with disabilities) had passed only a year or two before I went to college. There were debates in the field regarding appropriate education for students with significant disabilities.

One of my first big efforts after getting students mainstreamed into classes was to figure out ways for my students to participate in school activities and clubs, including sports. Out of this came the idea that Jay would become a manager for the football team. At that time, Walt Whitman High School was known for academic rather than gridiron success, but that didn't matter to Jay. His job as a football manager was to hand the players towels when they came off the field, and he took this role very seriously. In fact, every single player who came off that field got a towel, whether he needed one or not. Over the course of that season, Jay went to away games on the bus with the team; he often ate with the players in the cafeteria; and at the end of the season, at the football banquet, Jay received his football letter and jacket just like everyone else on the team.

These experiences impacted all of us in many ways. This was my first time moving outside of the comfort zone of my classroom and onto the football field. It required strong support of his family. Rud, I'm sure you well remember those cold Friday night games; and Amy and Kate, you must remember shopping for cool new clothes for Jay.

And it took members of the football team (a group not usually considered as highly sensitive high schoolers) to support Jay's success. It taught me the importance of making the effort, doing what I thought was right, and trusting that the community would be there to provide the safety net. It also raised the bar for me in terms of my vision of was possible for individuals with disabilities. I learned I didn't have to be there 100 percent of the time to support a student; and that others from the community (yes, even football players) could provide equally valuable support.

I know for Ann and Rud it also helped them to see a different future for Jay, one that focused on his full inclusion and participation in his community—doing what he liked best and not what we thought was best for him.

Finally, he made a difference by "paying it forward" to the young adults in high school that year. I particularly think about a young woman named Nikky who went on to become a special education teacher. I remember hearing from her several years ago about how her experiences with Jay and the other students in the class helped make that decision for her.

I even learned a little bit about Kansas University (KU) Jayhawk spirit. I remember one fine morning in March when Jay showed up in a t-shirt and hat with NCAA 1988 championship emblazoned upon it. Not knowing a single thing about what either NCAA or Jayhawks meant, I remember being puzzled by his appearance. It took me two years and only upon my arrival to KU to finally put that piece of the puzzle in place.

The transition to adult life in Lawrence for Jay was often difficult and full of trial and error. In so many ways, he was forging new ground in terms of what it meant to be fully included in the adult community.

He moved into his own home with the support of two KU students, Pat and Cory. They forged a friendship that expanded Jay's network within the KU community. Jay was initiated as an honorary member of the SAE fraternity and regularly attended meetings and don't forget the parties. He started to branch out into his community, ever expanding his circle of inclusion.

When I look out into the church, I am awed by the network of people here who were touched by Jay, including my husband. He met Jay on our second date at an event for advocates that included the late singer songwriter, Tom Hunter, debuting a song entitled, "It's Awesome to be Surrounded by People Who Aren't Sorry"—a song for and about Jay. As I recall, the lyrics were inspired by an observation Amy made about Jay's extensive circle of supports and friends. It's about providing the supports Jay needed to be a full contributing member of his community.

From these years, while not always easy, I most remember the lesson we learned of allowing JT to lead us down the right road. We didn't always know how to pay attention to his passion for his life to be a certain way until he made it loud and clear what he didn't like. Clearly, when you were around Jay, you could not just talk the talk; you had to walk the walk, and he was the trailblazer creating that path.

Nan Hunt, a long-time friend of Jay's, wrote after she heard the sad news: "Jay lived in such a way that the message of his life was very clear. He did not rush or hurry… Jay was Jay and that was that. Either you accepted him or you didn't, either way made no difference to him. He had accepted himself and unconditionally loved those around him. The wonderful thing about Jay was he did not define his life through ownership of things or worldly success. He simply touched lives. He did not possess them; he touched them, accepted them, and loved."

That very simple message of love and joy in how to live life with passion is one that I will try to hold onto in Jay's honor.

Postscript: Jay in Context— Public Policy, Our Profession, and Our Best Professor

There is no end to Jay's life, no closings. Death has removed him, his physical self, from us, but he lives in me still, as he does in Ann, Amy, and Kate.

On the seventh of each month, Ann and I go to his grave. Sometimes, we bring fortune cookies; sometimes, M&M candies, his favorites. Other days, I go there by myself, sometimes with gifts other than myself.

These visitations are compulsory: I can no more not do them than not breathe. They are equally life-giving, sources of remembrance, grief, and joy.

Writing, too, persists: Jay's death and my life, its subjects.

The psychological journey is, after all, the only one worth narrating.

Jay compelled us to take the journey, and he was its navigator through all the years. Ann, Amy, and Kate were inseparable companions on it.

Ann's and my trip intersected with most, if not all, of the major changes in policy and practice in the field of intellectual and related developmental disability—changes in which Ann and I had the honor to participate in rather significant ways. Because of Jay and Ann, I am a student of the human condition in a policy context. And because of Jay, Ann is the most authentic voice of all voices in the field of intellectual disability.

Amy is a social worker, expert in low-income housing, a graduate of the University of Kansas (B.S., M.S., both in social welfare administration) and now a doctoral student at the University of Chicago. Kate also is a graduate of the University of Kansas (B.A.) and of the University of San Diego (M.F.A.) and now an actress in New York City and teacher of theatre in its public schools and psychiatric hospitals. Their chosen professions reflect the impact Jay had on them—the pursuit of justice for those who have special challenges. As for the journey Ann and I have taken, it has been fulfilling in the extreme.

It was one thing for physicians at Johns Hopkins to recommend institutionalization. It would have been altogether another for them to recommend that we withdraw all life support to Jay. Indeed, Jay was not technologically dependent. Unlike other newborns, he was healthy. Yet the matter of withholding and withdrawing life support from newborns and others at the end of their lives has been a central policy issue for me.

Jay and I experienced the charity model—the "cap in hand" culture—when he attended the pre-school in Durham and then the private schools, Pine Harbor Nursery, in Rhode Island and Crystal Springs Nursery, in Massachusetts. In time, the charity model yielded to a rights model; both co-exist now (2010).

It is significant that Pine Harbor Nursery was operated by a religious order—significant because the charity model was, in many of its manifestations, theologically based. The interaction of charity, theology, and emerging (and now solid) rights-based response to the needs of families and their members with disabilities was hardly new and persists even now.

Ann and I have been rights-advocates while not in the least rejecting the spiritual and secular communities that dedicate themselves to individuals with disabilities. These models are not necessarily mutually exclusive.

I institutionalized Jay; I cannot say it in any other way. Yes, Pine Harbor and Crystal Springs were privately operated, but they were institutions nonetheless. They were not the horrific public institutions of the time, not at all. But they were unacceptable to Ann and me.

Ann and I brought Jay home to us and, even before doing so, co-authored our first publication. In it we argued for de-institutionalization. We have never stopped making that argument, but we have added two others to it. First, we have advocated for family support, and, next, for home- and community-based services.

Had there been sufficient family support and home and community based services when Jay was young, it may have been unnecessary for Jay to live with Cordelia Bethea or "go away to school" at Pine Harbor and Crystal Springs. Once Ann and I married, we were determined that we would create policy and practice that would make it possible for families who so wish to stay intact, with support.

When Jay failed in the behavior modification experiments at the Kennedy Institute in Baltimore, I learned much about consent and applied behavior modification. When I was on human rights committees of institutions in North Carolina and Ann was a member of the staff of an institution in Alabama, we both learned too much about aversive and punishing interventions. And when Jay was in the adult service system in Lawrence, we came face to face with the consequences of resistance to the pursuit of excellence and evidence-based interventions.

Our professional work has focused on the rights and realities of consent, regulation of placements, and interventions that are demonstrably ineffective, legally objectionable, and ethically noxious. At the same time, we have taught students, operated programs, and carried out research on how policy, families, and professionals can develop their capacities for effective, legal, and ethical interventions and support.

Jay was fortunate in many respects. Among them is that he was in the first cohort of students to have a right to a free appropriate public education. Ann and I have made that right a central part of our advocacy, research, and teaching, remembering in particular that segregation by disability and race were parts of Jay's life.

So much of Jay's quality of life depended upon how Amy and Kate understood him and responded to his disabilities. He shaped them profoundly. Ann is responsible for adapting a "family systems theory" to families affected by disability; both of us advocate that brothers and sisters need support, not just parents and the person with a disability.

Jay's inclusion into Chapel Hill, his fuller inclusion into Walt Whitman High School, and his eventual remarkable inclusion, as an adult, into Lawrence derived from our instincts against segregation, for integration, and for legal principles and practices that create community among those with and those without disabilities.

More than that, we have concluded that the joy quotient is the ultimate measure of the work families and professionals do together for a person with a disability. The enviable life that Jay had, and that other families and individuals affected by disability should have, results from humane policy, its effective implementation, and partnerships among professionals, families, and community members. Integration, partnership, and "giving away to the community"—creating an intentional family for the person with a disability, assuring genuine social security—are matters of law, practice, and ethics. These, too, are among our professional concerns.

We have been guided by understandings that Jay gave us: play from a position of strength, have great expectations, give choices and create the capacity to know and exercise choices, develop relationships and communal bonds, seek and embrace the positive contributions that people with disabilities make to us, and insist on their and our full citizenship, whether in work, residential living, or spiritual communities. These are tenets of our work, but, more, they are some of Jay's lessons to us.

As much as Jay's community support meant to him and us, there is no doubt but that he benefited greatly from entitlements under the Social Security Act and from the wise use of strategies to marshal and maximize private and public benefits simultaneously. We have been involved in advocacy to create home and community based services, preserve supplemental security income, and enlarge the choices available to individuals and families on how to use the medical insurance and supplemental income entitlements.

There is more—but these are the core issues of our professional life. Is there a theme to them? Yes, but not just one.

Because of Jay, we have rejected, and tried to persuade others, in policy and practice, to reject, stereotypes about disability, and we have sought policy, practice, and revision of cultural norms that limit because of stereotype.

And because of Jay, we have proclaimed that less able does not at all mean less worthy.

And, finally, because of Jay we radically accepted and joyously rejoiced in the life Jay brought to us—one shaped by the difference known as disability.

It is inappropriate for this chronicle about Jay to detail my and Ann's roles in these policy and practice matters. It is essential, however, for us to declare that, were it not for Jay, we would have not had any of those roles.

He was our best professor, a charter member of the vanguard that sought and attained huge reforms of policy, practice, and the professions, and an exemplar to those who have read our writings, heard our stories, and learned about him.

He was all that, but, of course, he was more, much more.

* * *

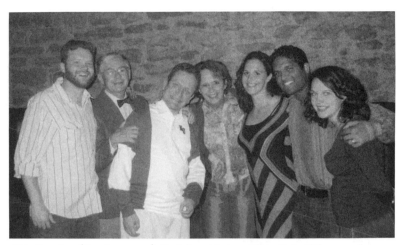

Chip Brookes (Kate's partner), Rud, Jay, 40, Ann, Kate, Rahul Khare, and Amy, 2007

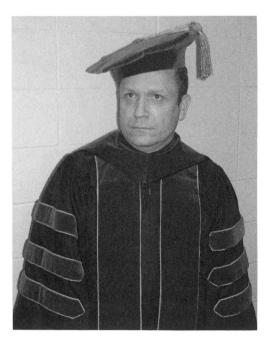

Jay, 40, his parents' best professor, in Rud's academic regalia, 2007

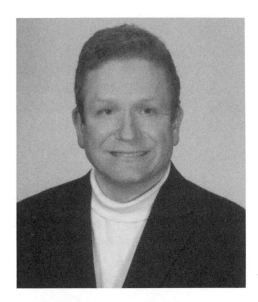

Jay, 41, as an honorary member of Kappa Sigma fraternity, University of Kansas, 2008

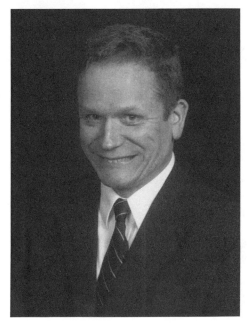

Jay, 41, Lawrence, Ks., 2008

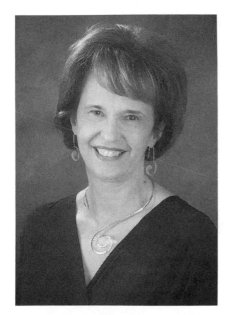

Ann, 2008

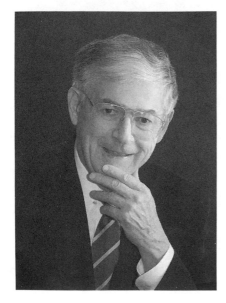

Rud, 2008

341

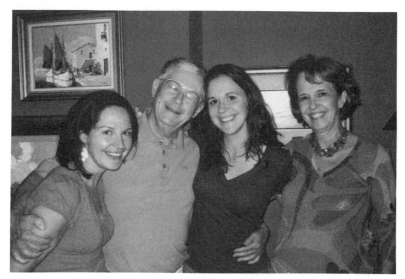

Amy, Rud, Kate, and Ann, Lawrence, Ks., 2010